Out of your
MIND
—AND—
into your
HEART

Using love energy
to heal your life

MARIE ROBERTS

Foreword by
Richard C. Miller, Ph.D.

THE CROSSING PRESS
FREEDOM, CALIFORNIA

For information on bulk purchases or group discounts for this and other Crossing Press titles, please contact our Special Sales Director at 800/777-1048, ext. 203.

www.crossingpress.com

Library of Congress Cataloging-in-Publication Data
Roberts, Marie, 1951-
  Out of your mind and into your heart : using love energy to heal your life / Marie Roberts.
    p. cm.
  ISBN 1-58091-110-2 (pbk.)
  1. Spiritual life.   I. Title.
BL624 .R6218 2001
291.4'4--dc21

                              2001042386

Advanced reader copy
0 9 8 7 6 5 4 3 2 1

Dedication

To the two who chose me as mother and taught me to give love a chance: Amy Moryl-Roberts and Seth Barton-Roberts. My heart recognized you before you were born.

Acknowledgments

This book is a reflection on the journey of a lifetime and was inspired by all the teachers and writers who encouraged me to look beyond intellect for the truth. They are too many to name, but I bow to them in gratitude. Thanks to Linda Urie, whose very presence is the reminder of another dimension and whose intuitive guidance led me to The Crossing Press. Thanks also to Elaine Gill for believing in this project from the moment the pages crossed her desk and for offering her impressive skills as editor and publisher. And, of course, my appreciation goes to the two children, Amy and Seth, who've opened my heart in their own unique ways, and to some dear friends who show me every day what love is all about. To Ann De Paolo, my biggest cheerleader; to Janet Jepsen, a long-time rock in my life's foundation; to Sigal Brier and Gudrun von Auenmueller for always being willing to go deep into Spirit with me; and to Sturgis Poorman, who never thinks I'm crazy, even when I am. And most of all to Spirit, whose activity in my life never ceases to amaze me.

Contents

FOREWORD By Richard C. Miller, Ph.D. 9

INTRODUCTION Confessions of a Recovering Intellectual 17

CHAPTER 1 We Want Love, but Where Is It
and How Do We Get It? 23

CHAPTER 2 The Heart: The Window of the Soul 39

CHAPTER 3 Embodying Love with Yoga, Body
Awareness, and Energy Balancing 57

CHAPTER 4 Meditation Practices for the
Devotionally Challenged 77

CHAPTER 5 Looking for Love in All the Right Places 105

CHAPTER 6 Choosing from Clarity 125

CHAPTER 7 The New Creation 143

Richard C. Miller, Ph.D.

The day will come when, after harnessing the wind, the waves and the tides, we shall harness for God the power of love. And on that day, for the second time in the history of the world, man will have discovered fire.

— Pierre Teillhard de Chardin

We live simultaneously in two worlds. We live with our feet planted in one world made up of solid and separate objects, which appear to exist independent of us. This is a world of duality in which we live informed by second-hand concepts that we take to be real. These concepts are stored in our bodymind as feelings, emotions, thoughts, beliefs, memories, and images. For instance, we were told a long time ago that we were born, that we have a body, that we are male or female and that we will die. We have accepted the legitimacy of these second hand beliefs which were based on the authoritative testimony of our ancestors. We may never have questioned their validity, but many people down through the ages have questioned their validity and have been astonished by what they uncovered when they finally experienced themselves through first hand knowing.

When we look with sincere innocence into these beliefs we hold to be true and respond with total honesty-without depending on our memory, which is based on second-hand information-we too will open into delight, wonder, and astonishment at the answers we come up with to such simple questions as, "How old do I really feel? Is my experience really that I have a body? What gender do I really feel myself to be? What is my true name?" These simple questions can move us beyond second hand concepts, beyond the world of duality, into experiencing a quite different reality that is not governed by the mind's past, but by the present moment, which is the realm of the heart. When we live in and from the heart, memory continues to function, but the mind no longer informs our experience. Instead, the heart informs the mind.

When we live informed by the heart, we discover that we are living in a parallel universe to the world of duality. Here, we live in a world of nondual, loving presence in which all objects are realized and perceived to be non separate projections of our own indivisible, nondual presence. In the world of the heart we experience the end of striving to become something other than what we already are. In the world of the heart, being is enough. Here, we find the heart's rest as we accept and welcome ourselves as we are. It is a relief to finally realize that we don't have to be different. In the heart's world, we are always being loved for who we are, not who we should be.

In a world of duality we strive to be more loving, kind, generous, and compassionate. But in the world of the heart, we discover our natural ground of being, in which we are love itself. We uncover our very nature and find it to be loving, kind, generous, and compassionate. These are the essential aspects of our being. When we live in the heart we don't experience separation. Here, there is only our self and everyone we see is realized to be 'I.' And when all we see is our self, who is there to hurt? Who then is there to tell a lie to, to be unkind to? There is only our self. Living in the heart brings an end to violence and deception. When we live in the heart we live selfishly: we are moved by our essential compassion and love to help our neighbor because we see that our neighbor is our self.

It can be disorienting a first when everyone we see is our self. It can be unsettling to contemplate that our striving to change our self is actually taking us away from being happy. Striving keeps us bound to our unhappiness. Striving is always for a future goal that lies forever 'out there.' When we stop striving and simply are, the mind grows quiet and we come to rest. It is important to note that in being, we do not become lethargic. The heart is divinely willful. Doing continues, but no longer from the attitude of trying to change our self. Simply stated, being is enough.

The nature of mind is to split that which is one into two. This is its inherent tendency. There's nothing wrong with this. It is just the way mind functions. Without the mind, we would not be able to conceptualize a cup to drink from, visualize a chair to sit in, or experience a separate 'other' with whom to have an intimate relationship. Our ability to live in the world of mind allows us to function as individuals and manipulate a world of separate objects. But separation comes with a hefty price tag. Separation and fear co-arise. They are not disparate movements. When we live only from the perspective of being separate individuals, we experience our lives filled with suffering, anxiety, and fear. And while we may try all kinds of remedial action, trying to bring an end to suffering, anxiety, and fear without solving the accompanying problem of separation is tantamount to rearranging the furniture on the Titanic. While any change may look good for a while, it provides no lasting resolution to the problem at hand. In order to bring an end to suffering, we must resolve the dilemma of feeling separate.

Our ability to bring an end to suffering depends on our capacity to examine our own lives. No external or internal repair ultimately works. Our ability to live in this world of duality while welcoming its various movements of sensation, feeling, emotion, and thought, provides the gateway we are looking for to enter this other wondrous world of loving presence where we feel whole, healed, and healthy. When we accept our self as we are, when we unflinchingly realize that our suffering rises out of our feeling alienated and separate from our self, we become vulnerable, open, and respectful for everything we feel and think and do. We no longer blame others, but see our own expectations that are clouding our vision. We no longer judge others for the way we feel, but experience our own longing to connect and share our self intimately with our self and with others.

To live our humanness is to experience joy and suffering. To live from our heart is to enter the domain of peace and loving kindness and the timeless reality of transcendent being. To live our presence and our humanness are not separate movements. They are one. We must understand that any attempt to rid ourselves of our humanness in order to become enlightened gives rise to suffering. What we fundamentally are is not dependent upon changing circumstances. However, exploring what does come and go opens us to experiencing our underlying, changeless, heartfelt presence in which all coming and going arises. Separation heals when our hearts are open to what is. By feeling the places in ourselves we have judged, compassion and loving kindness naturally arise. Paradox operates at every turn.

Being open to our self with deep trust and reverence facilitates healing. While we must be willing to face our self, by our self, community is a vital component in healing into the loving heart. Our wounds are the entry points for love, which takes us beyond separation and suffering. Community facilitates healing by supporting our moving into, rather than away from our experiences of separation. In community, as with self, we do not analyze or attempt to change. Instead our stories of limitation and separation are welcomed. In welcoming there is no prescription for being other than we are. And when we are open without expectation, what is welcomed ultimately empties into its underlying nature, which is unbounded, loving presence, the open, vulnerable heart.

Our defects are the ways that glory gets manifested.
Whosoever sees clearly what's diseased in himself
begins to gallop on the way...
Don't turn your head.
Keep looking at the bandaged place.
That's where the light enters you.
And don't believe for a moment
that you're healing your self.

-Rumi, Coleman Barks, The Essential Rumi

In Out of Your Mind and Into Your Heart, Marie Roberts opens us to her personal exploration in moving out of her mind and into her heart. She shares with us both intimate details of her own journey into awakening, as well as various ways and means that have helped her and countless others walk this path. Her book is an invitation for us to come into contact within ourselves and with that, which is most intimately playful and loving. Marie shows us that love will never be found in the past or the future, which is the mind. Love is alive only in this present moment. When we awaken into the heart we awaken to this present moment-to the now. While altars may be set with many adornments, the true altar is the heart that is tender, vulnerable, open, and welcoming. The heart that is on fire can't wait. The heart, your heart, truly craves an intimacy that heals all separation. And it wants it now. The heart knows the truth that it needs to tell in order to open into the world of the precious and loving presence that we truly are. Marie's invitation is for us to no longer postpone the inevitable, which is our full opening into the waiting arms of the heart.

Richard C. Miller
Sebastopol, CA

Richard Miller, Ph.D. has spent his life studying wisdom approaches to meditation and psychology as pathways to freedom. He has published widely in the field and leads retreats throughout the U.S. and Canada. He was co-founder of The International Association of Yoga Therapists and the founding editor of The Journal of IAYT. Richard is also a clinical psychologist with practices in San Rafael and Sebastopol, California.

CONFESSIONS OF A RECOVERING INTELLECTUAL

As one who lived in her head for the first forty years or so of her life, gratitude for my own transformation leads me to accompany you on this journey to the heartland. It is easier to be me now, and perhaps you are wondering how it can be easier to be you. Maybe you're coming at life from the opposite direction, from feeling rather than from intellect, but that doesn't mean that life is more fun for you, and it doesn't mean you're coming from your heart. We can be stuck in our heads or in our feelings, out of balance on either end of the seesaw.

Those buffeted by feelings may cast reason to the wind, following emotions into alien and even, at times, dangerous territory. In my twenty-five years as a spiritual guide, I have met people who are on the verge of destroying themselves or others because they react compulsively from their gut-level emotions. I have met people of great compassion who are doing little to remedy the evils they lament when they look around or turn on the evening news. They are so overwhelmed by emotion that they become immobilized.

If, on the other hand, you are coming as I did from a tendency to over-analyze, your handicap is supported by the culture where the ability to collect, sort, and analyze data is prized. As children, few of us were rewarded for experiencing and expressing our feelings. On the other hand, we were given high marks for the number of facts we could remember and repeat. If we came from emotionally arid or violent homes, there was even more incentive to deny our feelings. Feeling less meant you hurt less. Many of us learned early on to rationalize, rather than to live our reality.

As adults, whether in the past we avoided or overindulged our feelings, we probably live our lives presently at a frantic pace. Our inability to act appropriately shows, for instance, when we stick to a self-imposed five-year plan long after it stops suiting our needs. A professor I know wonders why he cannot write his post-doctoral research papers, even though he recognizes that he's following a course of action which he has lost enthusiasm for. It seemed right for him when he finished the Ph.D. years ago. Now he suffers from undiagnosed physical symptoms and a painful personal life as he struggles to remain true to his plans. "But I'd love to write a novel," he admits with a sigh. His self-control may be killing him. Others may be so caught up in the myriad details of everydayness that life becomes merely a series of out-of-control moments, exhibiting no sense of direction whatsoever. "I can't go to graduate school now," rues one talented would-be women's advocate who manages a large home. "I never know when I'll be hosting a dinner for my husband's colleagues."

We veer from one extreme to the other. We either make a desperate attempt to control everything and everybody or we abdicate any personal responsibility. "Life hurts," we say. And the underlying message may be: "If I'm hurting this much, don't expect me to be sorry if you're hurting, too. In fact, your pain validates my own experience." Our ability to empathize becomes impaired. "Life is tough," we say to ourselves and to everybody around us.

I said that a lot. And life had been tough for me. My father was addicted as much to rage as he was to alcohol. He bragged he would rather have his three daughters fear him than love him. He wasn't confusing the two emotions, nor did he even bother to try to convince us that the abuse was for our own good. Violence in our house was a way of life, and my mother's own anger and fear kept her from offering what could have been a compensatory softness. In fact, I can't remember any softness in my childhood years.

Keeping the family secret meant we were allowed very little interaction with the outside world except for school and church. As a Roman Catholic, I went to parochial school for the first three grades and did find some solace in dimly lit sanctuaries with flickering candles, heavy with incense. But the God I met there seemed far away from me and He came with a set of rules that did nothing to blur my already hardened edges.

The only asset I could count on was my intelligence—I excelled in school. This earned me approval and kindness from teachers and helped me develop a sense of my own worth. Additionally, since my parents saw their children as extensions of themselves, any honors I received staved off their wrath for the brief time they basked in reflected glory.

I was not a happy child, and it shows in almost every photograph taken of me. But I was an intelligent child, and that gave me hope. Reading was the only escape allowed, so I made numerous trips to the public library, bringing home armfuls of novels which I almost inhaled. Through them I lived lives far different from my own.

I could have had many friends if my parents hadn't frowned on any socializing outside of school, so I had to be satisfied with doing well and well I did. After high school, I worked my way through college and two graduate programs at the same time, and in addition I supported myself with a variety of jobs, scholarships, and assistant-ships. Drawn to life's depths, I nevertheless kept depth at bay by making it my chosen field of study. Philosophy, the-ology, spirituality, psychology—I took degrees with honors in all of them and was teaching at a college when I was twenty-four years old.

Still, it hurt to be me. At my core, I believed that life was the way my parents saw it. And because I believed it, so it was. On a peripheral level, I could tell people were attracted to me. However, I felt isolated, and so I was. I married more than once for what I assumed was love. However, I failed to bond with my husbands. I didn't go into the relationships with any expectation that my emotional needs would be met. I didn't even know what my emotional needs were.

Making career choices was far simpler. I was absolutely sure of myself. Based on intuition, I made good career choices, accepting or rejecting without guilt various credentials, titles, and positions. I started a second Master's degree before I had finished the first. And after two graduate degrees, I was able to drop out of the Ph.D. program I was on the verge of completing because I was eager to do more hands-on work with people. Drawn to the Protestant ministry, I was soon ordained. I worked very hard and made appropriate decisions almost without thinking.

Most of my other, more personal, decisions were made from a list of shoulds and oughts far removed from any sense of my own well-being. My leisure activities, friendships, relationships, and marriages did not for the most part repeat the violence of my childhood. For that I count my blessings. I have seen the devastation that such a legacy can leave in its wake. However, there was a lot of emotional harshness and hurt in my personal choices, and my soul died a little more each day. I knew it but didn't know what to do about it. My relationships had no juice in them, no joy, no shared purpose. Brainpower had helped me survive, but brainpower alone could not help me thrive. It could not teach me how to love and be loved. I knew instinctively that

I could not erase that emotional hole by analyzing it, but I also knew that I couldn't fill it with people, substances, or things. Neither head nor gut could heal me. The answer to my emotional dilemma had to be spiritual. Just knowing that, however, did not make everything right. I had explored theologies about God, but I did not yet know how to embrace the Sacred.

In the years since, I have found what was missing. Sometimes, little by little, sometimes by leaps and bounds, life changed me. Or you can say that I changed my life. I had help, lots of help. Tools, techniques, and teachers that my analytical mind had previously found intriguing, but unconvincing, began to shape my thoughts and emotions. I found my heart.

Reality feels very different when processed through the heart. Now, for me, rebirth is neither an academic theory nor part of a fundamentalist religious creed. It is an every-day occurrence. It can be for you, too. Antoine de Saint-Exupery said it well in *The Little Prince.* "Here is my secret, a very simple secret. It is only with the heart that one can see rightly; what is essential is invisible to the eye."

CHAPTER 1

WE WANT LOVE, BUT WHERE IS IT AND HOW DO WE GET IT?

In the limited and painful circumstances of my childhood, I eagerly devoured books from the library that helped me to picture other realities. These books helped me flesh out ideas that would otherwise have remained just theories. Beauty and kindness, for instance, were just words to me, attractive words to be sure, but concepts rather than experiences. Finding them lived out in the context of a story made them that much more real. I could imagine them in action, seeing in my mind's eye how they played out in the lives of actual or fictionalized characters. I was thereby inspired to include beauty and kindness in my life.

It was with the same rapt attention that I listened to the lyrics of songs on the radio. I liked the melodies, but I needed the words. They told me stories and helped me picture new ways of feeling. (To this day, much as I love certain classical pieces, music without lyrics doesn't hold my interest for long.) The way the words were sung also affected me. A good singer could remind me of emotions I knew I had, but was not free to express.

When I was seven or eight years old I remember asking myself why most of the songs I listened to had something to do with love. Whether the love mentioned in the song is celebrated or lamented, whether the song appeals to what is sentimental, romantic, or cosmic, it's still all about love. Love is what makes us want to sing. These songs speak to our joys, our sorrows, our yearnings. We want love, but what is it and how do we get it?

From St. Francis of Assisi, to Ann Landers, to any number of contemporary spiritual writers, the advice is the same: If you are seeking love, be the lover. Come from fullness rather than from need. You can only attract what you already carry within you and are demonstrating to the world. "All well and good," you respond. "But how can I love when I have never been loved, or have never been loved in the right way?" Or you may say, "How can I be the lover when there is no one around to whom I can give all this love inside of me?"

These are very intelligent questions, but they are not productive. Ask them and nothing changes, and change is what you're after or you wouldn't be asking the questions in the first place. This kind of question invites speculation, self-pity, or anger rather than transformation. It is based on flawed assumptions about the nature of love that spring from our culture's flawed assumptions about the nature of reality itself.

For the past several hundred years, science has presumed to define reality. Prior to the scientific age, religion did that for us. Now neither seems adequate to the task. So we turn to a spirituality that illumines both while eschewing the dogmatism of each. Spirituality has to do with finding the essence—of the person, of the world, of the cosmos, and ultimately of reality itself.

Christian spiritual tradition, for example, seeks to introduce us to Ultimate Reality in its scriptures. "God is Love," proclaims the First Letter of John in the Bible. Notice that the line does not read, "God acts lovingly," "God loves creation," or even "God is loving," although that is often the meaning we see in it. The Biblical statement as it stands indicates an equal relationship between God and Love. God and Love are two sides of the same equation, sharing an identity on either side of the verb. So we are not talking about God's attitude or behavior, but the nature of God. The nature of divinity is love. In other words, the very essence of God, the Reality from which we spring and in which we swim, is love.

Monotheistic religions have used the word "God" to describe the source and nature of reality, but the word God can be misused and misunderstood. It sets up another entity in our lives, one far grander and more mysterious than we can comprehend. Communication between us and God seems to occur across a great chasm and with much fear and trembling on our side. Something about this picture of God does not ring true for the 21st century and, indeed, has never completely rung true for many of us. It is a picture alien to Eastern traditions, and one which Western theologians have been struggling to reframe for centuries.

Martin Buber, a Jewish scholar, called God "Thou." In true intimacy, each person is a Thou to the other, and the sense of otherness begins to melt. God is the primary source of that experience, the Thou to which we all can relate intimately. Paul Tillich, a Lutheran, said that the Divine could not be described as a being, but as Being Itself. He also made it clear that, while God cannot be described as a person, God is indeed personal. Statements like these intrigued me in graduate school and gave me hope. I was not willing to discard my awareness of the sacred because of a flawed description of God.

In seeking a practical way to live joyously from the heart, let's move beyond theoretical abstraction and simplistic fundamentalism, whether we find either in religion or in science. Let's instead ask the basic question. How can we change our lives? There is an answer that validates our own experience while inviting us to transform it. It is a spiritual answer that resonates with the best of religion and science. The answer is energy or vibration.

I remember an afternoon in third grade science class when the teacher pointed to the desks, chairs, and blackboard in the room and told us that, while they looked solid and felt solid, they were actually composed of moving molecules. I looked around. We all stared at our hands in wonder. Nothing was as it seemed! This revelation lent a kind of fluidity and possibility to the world. However, we were never encouraged to ponder the wonder of all this or connect it with the lesson on religion we had earlier in the day. (This was a parochial school and our teacher was a Roman Catholic nun.) And as we progressed through elementary and high school, we were never reminded of this truth about this unseen movement in seemingly solid objects.

Think about it. All of us were taught at one time or another that reality is not what it looks like to the naked eye. However, we must act as if only what is directly and physically observable is real. I had to live in the delusion of solidity and lack of motion in order to move through the educational system, but the kernel of truth remained like a buried treasure. What the new physics is rediscovering is the sense of wonder that began for me in that third grade science class.

Our bodies are not what they seem. However, that information has not sunk in for most of us. Although we say that our bodies are alive, we tend to treat them as if they were dead. Solid to the touch and genetically programmed, they seem to us to be a closed system, utterly predictable when fed and watered. When we get sick or hurt in some way, we're baffled and look to medical doctors to fix us or give us a prognosis as to how long our bodies will continue to function. But healers have always known what Western medicine has not always remembered. Our bodies are solid to the touch, yes, but hardly impermeable. Matter is permeable or impermeable, light or dense, depending upon the frequency at which its molecules vibrate. We ourselves are conscious vibrations. We can choose to move to a higher frequency.

And so we come to the chakra system of ancient India. (The Sanskrit word *chakra* means a wheel.) Chakras are whirling eddies of energy. I first heard the word in a world religion class in graduate school and dismissed it, thinking it was simply a part of a theoretical system that had very little to do with my life. Not until my own heart chakra made itself known did I remember what I had learned years before.

There are seven major chakras with the heart chakra at the center. "Where are they?" you may legitimately ask, especially if you are as skeptical as I was. "I don't see them on my skin, and they are surely not hiding somewhere inside me. They don't show up on an X-ray." Chakras are real, but they are energetic realities. They are not found on or in the physical body, because they are part of the ongoing process of creating that physical body. They are the points at which the creation process is most likely to flow smoothly or to get stuck.

For instance, we are meant to allow creation to happen in such a way that we are grounded—in strong lower body parts such as legs and hips—and have an emotional sense of our own entitlement to be here on the planet. But that does not always happen. For a variety of reasons, some people's lower body parts do not function well. This affects their emotional experience of being present in a stable way. The reverse may also be true. For a variety of reasons some people may lack the emotional resources that enable them to feel entitled to be in their life situation and well placed there. The lower physical body will probably feel some effects from this sense of insecurity: very heavy and burdensome or fragile and beset by illness or accident. The first chakra at the base of the spine (you can visualize yourself sitting on it), is the site of this energy conversion. Chakras are where emotional blocks can become physical symptoms or physical symptoms can turn into emotional issues. So there are issues and symptoms for each chakra, although they are interrelated. When one wheel sticks it affects the functioning of all the wheels.

The second chakra is at the pelvis. It processes issues of sexuality, creativity, pleasure, and guilt. The third is at the solar plexus and deals with matters of personal power. The fourth is at the heart. We will discuss it later in greater detail. It processes the ability to love and relate. The fifth is at the throat and has to do with self-expression and communication. The sixth is at the third eye in the middle of the forehead. It is our seat of imagination and intuitive knowledge. The seventh is on the crown of the head. It opens us up to inspiration, faith, and a deeper connection to all of life. The issues of each chakra may be addressed by a combination of physical, mental, emotional, and spiritual techniques. There is no right or wrong place to begin healing.

As the lower and upper chakras begin to open more, you will feel their effects in the heart chakra.

Each chakra vibrates as a sound and color. From the base of the spine to the crown, the chakra colors begin with red and go up to become orange, yellow, green, blue, indigo, and violet, sometimes with a white light pouring out from that violet. How does your self-image change when you picture yourself as a walking rainbow? Ponder that when you are feeling low.

To return to the question we asked at the beginning of the chapter: "How can I love when I have not been loved adequately or if there is no worthy object of my affections?" The heart chakra is one of the seven conduits for a life energy that is always ready to flow. Its functionality can be damped, blocked, or hidden, but can never be truly lost. The blockage may have happened when you were in a threatening or restrictive situation, and in order to cope with your own vulnerability, you shut down. My work as a spiritual director has shown me that fear is what keeps most of us from moving along. You may have everything on the outside. You may have looks, family, money—whatever—and still be very fearful inside. You may not feel entitled to what you have, or you may feel that you are entitled to much more than you will ever get, or you may be afraid that it is all going to be taken away from you. That's not necessarily what you say, but behavior and attitude give you away.

The chakras whirl when they are happy, and we dance to their rhythm. When I notice that I have stopped dancing and am sinking into depression, anger, restlessness, or hyperactivity, it's good to ask myself, "What am I afraid of?" This is first chakra stuff, although its effects can be noticed anywhere along the energy pathway. For instance, you may be unhappy because you do not speak your mind very often. This is a congestion at the throat, the fifth chakra. You can work on this in many ways, from voice lessons, to public speaking, to small attempts at making yourself known at home or at work. But it is also wise to ask the underlying question, "What am I afraid of?" This can be the best question for those who appear the least afraid, that is — for those who live in their heads. These people may look like they've got everything under control because their actions are so deliberate, or because they like to appear optimistic all the time. In either case, the first chakra needs to be dealt with. It doesn't matter whether our style is to get stuck in the first chakra or to live as far away from it as possible. Both attitudes are unconscious reactions to fear, and love and fear do not live in the same place.

The same First Letter of John in the Bible tells us that "perfect love casts out fear." Those who have become attuned to the vibrations of the heart space will find themselves able to love even those who hate them. This is where true faith leads. But as we begin the journey it is wise to keep in mind the statement as it can be reversed: "Overwhelming fear casts out love." So don't dismiss your fears without acknowledging them. At a very formative stage of your life, you may have known people who confused fear and love, people whose neediness drove them to proclaim their love for those who were hurting them physically or emotionally. It is important for you to understand that the people who chose to stay in such relationships were not doing so out of love, but out of fear. The fear may have been of the abusive person(s) or of what life would be like without them. This is first chakra congestion. It is insecurity masquerading as relationship. You received a message, based on a lie, that you may be wasting precious energy trying to embody. Don't feel bad. In the past you did whatever you needed to do to survive. Give yourself a pat on the back. But this is now, and what you did then to cope probably no longer serves you. You can change things by making the activation of the heart chakra a part of your daily life. Of course that means you will have to monitor your fears regularly, because those fears want to keep you from changing.

You can monitor your fears through recognizing the particular issues and symptoms that arise from time to time in all the chakras. However, by making the heart chakra a priority, you can literally clear a pathway for love. What is required is the desire to access heart energy and the decision to do so. Granted, this may be an easier desire to have and an easier decision to implement once you have had a healthy firsthand experience of loving and being loved. (Although, strange as it may seem to those of us coming from troubled childhoods, I have known quite a few people from loving, functional families who've had just as much trouble as I've had finding and keeping love.) Don't give up.

Just remember that love is the essence of all that is. Indeed, it is the very power that draws each group of molecules together into meaningful form. The ability to experience it is inherent to the human condition. We are all capable of finding love.

The following chapters include some exercises and tools for accessing heart energy. Maybe you are dissatisfied with where you are now, but are you ready to begin the work? See if you can cultivate a more neutral attitude toward whatever happened to you in the past. Curiosity is a good place to start. Set aside assumptions and make believe you have no idea why your life has unfolded as it has. Here a little psychotherapy can be an asset. You want to explore your feelings around certain events in the past so that you can experience them and let them go. What you do not want is to get so used to the process of telling your story over and over that you begin to believe that *you* are your story.

I once taught fourth grade in a private school and remember a moody little girl who never seemed happy. One day I corrected her on something she did or said. She looked up at me, crossed her arms in front of her chest, and said petulantly, "That's just the way I am and that's the way I'm always going to be." Her self-image was already carved in stone. Her script was written. It's hard to open to the possibility of each moment when you are tied into a script.

I used to advise my women clients who were going out on dates that it was a good sign when a man revealed that he was in long-term therapy. I have since reconsidered, having noticed that sessions with a therapist you have seen for a very long time can function more as reinforcement for your present behavior than as a catalyst for change. Hour-long conversations with someone who is paid to listen and whose responses are almost predictable are very attractive to a person on the edge of narcissism. It takes a very capable therapist to be effective after that length of time. A smart therapist understands the futility of trying to wean such a client away from a life script that isn't working, but may be reluctant to end the relationship for a variety of reasons. So, while counseling can be a great tool, it is not in itself evidence that you are ready to change your life. You do not want to attach yourself to your story; you want to feel it, claim it, make peace with it, reframe it if necessary, and then disengage from it.

The addiction to drama is perhaps the basic addiction. Wise spiritual teachers have advised me to step away from the drama and get out of my own way. Like many people, I stayed in places, relationships, jobs—whatever—longer than I needed to because I thought that every story had to play itself out, even when I was suffering adverse effects (perhaps especially when I was suffering adverse effects). After all, childhood had taught me that growth was about suffering. But little successes in seeing things differently and doing things differently led to my being able to make positive choices more often.

I knew how far I had when "my" daytime soap came to a close. For more than twenty years I had watched *Another*

World—compulsively during my graduate school days, more casually afterwards. Still the characters in that soap were my friends, and when it went off the air, it was hard to believe that they were gone for good. I toyed with the notion of following the leading characters who were able to make the transition to other soaps, but talked myself out of doing so. It wasn't about the stories themselves. After all, Charles Dickens' novels were first serialized in the popular press of his day because people love an ongoing story. Sometimes we just need a break from the daily grind. But my attachment to this form of entertainment had become more than a harmless diversion. It mirrored my willingness to forsake clarity for melodrama, especially in matters of the heart. I'd be picturing "happily ever after" instead of paying attention to what was actually going on. And I wasn't above using television to distract myself whenever I was on the verge of discovering the truth. So it took a while to notice that my romantic relationship had developed its own dys-functional story line. Then it took another few months to end things. After I did, I realized that I no longer needed the brand of romance offered by the soaps. I also decided that my time and energy could be put to better use.

There have been years when I struggled to make sense of my own history. It was probably necessary. My mind wanted to analyze all the nuances and details of my past and I had many questions. Why had I been so hurt as a defense-less child? Were there people who had an easier time of growing up? Why was life so unfair? Was my job in life to identify with and save the oppressed because I had known oppression firsthand? If so, how could I ever enjoy myself with a clear conscience? I finally got to the place where I could see that I had developed a tremendous strength in dealing with adversity. However, it was still hard to let go of my outrage over the injustice of it all and stop blaming those who had so wronged me. I had made the best of a bad situation, but that still did not make the situation right.

What happened to me was not right. Perhaps what happened to you was not right either. Now, as an adult, when I have the chance to prevent the abuse of any person by another, I will try to do that. Those who are vulnerable deserve our protection. I deserved more protection than I received. But it was doing me no good to constantly interpret my own story from the standpoint of what I deserved but did not receive. Nor was it helping to believe that because I did not receive protection, I must be unworthy in some way or that my whole life must manifest the awareness of suffering.

An old Buddhist story tells of a woman who went to the village sage after her child died. He gave her the task of going from door to door, saying he could help her once she had located the home that death had not visited. Of course, she could find none. That put her situation in perspective so that real healing could begin. When we are mired in self-pity and bitterness, no matter how well-deserved, we are only adding to our own misery. Carlos Castaneda in *Journey to Ixtlan* quotes his shamanic teacher, Don Juan, as saying:

"We either make ourselves miserable, or we make ourselves strong. The amount of work is the same." We can use our energy wastefully or productively. Sad things happen to us over the course of a lifetime. Misery, however, is an attitude, a choice. So is joy.

Beginning to view your own story impassively, with curiosity, is a good first step because it creates some distance between you and it. My life has become much easier since I have learned to use three sentences frequently and with some humor. The sentences each contain three words, and each sentence begins with the letter I: I love you, I don't know, and Isn't that interesting. The first speaks for itself, the second speaks to my recovery from intellectualism and my relief at not needing to have all the answers. The third is about creating a healthy distance between how I experience an event and how it originates. My ego wants to take every perceived slight personally. However, I must admit that most of what happens around me is not about me at all. This includes things said or done by those near and dear to me. Of course, I will not willingly allow myself to be hurt by someone else. But I will not flatter myself by imagining that I am necessarily the reason for that behavior. Your husband or wife, your child, your co-worker, the neighbor next door—they are all individuals living many different realities each day. Most of their attention is focused on trying to cope. You may trigger a negative reaction in any one of them, but that probably says more about them than you. I've learned to breathe through an initial affront, saying to

myself, "Isn't that interesting," thus allowing the dust to settle and the real nature of our relationship to emerge.

When you have been truly victimized at a vulnerable
point in your life, it is part of the healing process to
acknowledge it, and to feel your feelings about what happened and who hurt you. However, the more importance
you attach to your identity as a victim, the more likely it is
that victimhood will become a permanent state. Chances
are that you will be picked on, insulted, and hurt often, or
that you will turn into someone who does those things to
others. There is big truth in the statement that what we
expect to happen, we draw to ourselves. It is important to
really get that when we ponder some of life's most devastat-
ing experiences. We may not feel we have chosen those
experiences, but we can certainly decide what our attitude
toward them will be.

Once we have chosen to move beyond the place of vic-
timization, many more choices open up. The heart is the
beacon that draws love and light to us. Choose to move a
little distance away from your life's drama, choose to view
more events with benevolent humor, choose to make use of
some of the tools and techniques offered in the following
chapters. My hunch is that you will begin to tune into the
power of your heart energy and make a difference in yourself and the world around you.

CHAPTER 2

THE HEART:
THE WINDOW OF THE SOUL

When I revealed part of my life journey to a counselor with psychic abilities, she commented, "I can see the stone in your heart dissolving." She meant that the place where energy was blocked had formed a mass. It was true—I was blocked early on when I was a child, but now the life force was able to course through the part of me that had shut down.

I knew it was happening, but it was wonderful to have her confirmation. It felt like the thawing of an ice-crusted creek when a warm spring is underway. If you can read energetic patterns, you will experience in an instant the blurring of harsh edges and the resulting fluidity, just as clearly as if over a period of several months you had the opportunity to observe that icy creek crack open slowly so that the water could flow easily once more.

I do not yet have the gift of "seeing" the energetic flow with such detail and clarity. However, I have found that the more I pay attention to sensation—what I can physically see, hear, smell, taste, and touch—the more non-physical data I pick up. So often we are reading energy, although we don't admit to ourselves that that's what we're doing. For instance, I remember one morning years ago. I was walking across the campus of the university where I served as chaplain, when a woman I knew only in passing came out of one of the graduate dorms. Something about her face and posture struck me as troubled, and I asked how she was. "Oh, just fine," she replied cheerfully. I didn't have time to probe further. I was on my way to a meeting, and, more important, I had only my fleeting impression to go on. An hour later I saw her tearfully pouring her heart out to someone who had stopped to listen. I did not intrude, of course, for she was obviously being well cared for. I realized I had subliminally registered her pain, but had not taken my first impressions seriously. I had let myself be persuaded by her intentionally upbeat response. It was a big lesson for me. In those days it took hard data to convince me to trust my intuition. The incident changed me—it provided me with enough data to trust my subliminal impressions in the future. My transformation may have already begun, but it received a big boost that particular day.

Please don't get the idea that I am downplaying the value of the rational mind. I am blessed with a high level of intelligence. Book learning comes easy for me, so does strategic planning. I can usually figure out what is going on in a complex situation, and I am not averse to masterminding a plan so that things turn out my way. Because I can do these things, it is tempting to do them often. It is also easy to believe that my answers lie in books and that other sources are not important. Such beliefs complicate my life unnecessarily. Meticulous planning can turn into a desperate attempt to control my environment, including the people around me, which makes neither them nor me happy.

One advisor called this set of capacities "my general." He suggested that I allow my soul to be the general's commander-in-chief. I had explained to him that I wanted a less taxing way of life and wondered aloud whether I would have to give up using my brain entirely. "Of course not," he said reassuringly. "You have a wonderful brain. What you want to do is to use your brain in the service of your spirit instead of the other way around." I breathed a sigh of relief, for I had been harboring fears that in order to be spiritual I would have to get a little stupid. And that prospect was not at all appealing.

Perhaps we are all inclined to see the people who dedicate themselves to the spiritual path as somewhat naive. Since they know their allegiance is to a higher power, they may come across as simple to the powers that be, those pseudo powers that govern our desires to look good and succeed at any cost. We forget that spiritual teachers have used their keen intelligence so that they could make sense of the truths they experienced and bring their message to others. The Buddha moved out of his father's palace in order to experience life fully. He confronted all sorts of natural and supernatural peril and matched wits with the most clever minds. His enlightenment was not the result of dumb luck. It was a calculated experiment. He was as successful as his father would have wanted him to be, but he had a different goal. Jesus told his followers to be "innocent as doves" but also "wise as serpents." He told them not to linger with people who did not respect them. He himself did the same. When followers were overwhelming him with their needs, when disgruntled representatives of the religious or political establishment were haranguing him, he would sometimes hop in a boat and row to the other shore. He could have died many times before his final breath. At a crucial point, he allowed himself be taken by the Romans (for, indeed, this is the voluntary, sacrificial nature of his murder). If he had fled, he would have compromised his truth and invalidated the meaning of his life. Reading the gospels with eyes wide open, we can see the genius working through him.

The point is not to deny our intellectual capacities, but to put them in proper perspective. We describe people who rely solely on rationality when making a decision as "left-brained" and those who act spontaneously as "right-brained." Neither is better or worse than the other. From the physiological standpoint, left and right are two halves of a whole and are not intended to act independently of each other. When we refer to the energetics of the body, we focus on the process of balancing these tendencies. The process is about moving excess weight from the ends of the seesaw toward the middle. In the chakra system, that center is the heart.

Let's use a concrete example.

It is fine to live in the country; but unless there is a road or expressway between your home and your workplace, you are trapped and unproductive. It is fine to work in the city; but unless you can get home at twilight for a meal and relaxation, you are trapped and overextended. If the body is like a map, the heart would be the location of the expressway's most crucial bottleneck.

It is fine to experience the lower chakra feelings related to your basic human drives (security, pleasure, power), but unless these drives can be brought up through the heart, they will ensnare you. It is fine to experience the upper chakra's emphasis on communication, knowledge, and inspiration; but unless they can be brought down through the heart, you are left dangling in mid air. We all know people whom we would call either stuck (caught in the lower chakras) or spacey (caught in the higher chakras). People who live primarily from the waist down can be addicted to (or terrified of) anger, control, or lust, but they can also play at seeming well grounded. However, being in a rut is not the same as being grounded. It means being mired in a routine designed to mask the experience of fear and insecurity. People who live primarily from the neck up can be overly intellectual, but can also play at seeming highly conscious. However, being an airhead is not the same as being a sage. Airheads lack the ability to appropriately embody their ideas and intuitions.

The heart is where all human capacities can be integrated and put to good use. If there is no jam, traffic can move.

If there is no ice, creek water can flow. If there is no stone, life can flourish. This is something we seem to know intuitively. How interesting that, in an age that treats reality as just an ever-expanding data base, we are inundated with heart-shaped images.

We sit in front of our computers rather than venturing out to shake the hand of another flesh-and-blood human being. We work 16-hour days, oblivious to the personal relationships disintegrating around us. Yet when we do get out and sit across the table from an actual person, we may notice that the restaurant menu sports little hearts next to some of its entrees. And words like "heartsmart" and "hearthealthy" have become part of our working vocabulary. Of course, the symbols and words may simply refer to a concern for physical health. Heart disease is a major concern for a good portion of the population, as is cancer. But I wonder whether heart disease is a physical reminder of a more pervasive problem. What are the deeper needs that this concern for physical well-being manifests?

Since ancient times the word heart has been used to refer to the fullest expression of the human being. When used metaphorically, it represents the whole drive and attitude of a person. It has always been natural, for instance, when inquiring about people's opinions to ask them to speak from their hearts. The Hebrew scriptures are full of such references. They tell of those who harden their hearts against God or God's people. For example, this was said of Pharaoh when he refused to set the Hebrew people free. In the Bible, living according to divine intention is described as serving God with all one's heart, and experiencing a transformation in outlook is referred to as being given a new or clean heart. Hearts are soft or stony, they lament, or they rejoice. Of course. But why should this be so? The study of anatomy was not very sophisticated in those days, so it is safe to say that most ancient writers were not making reference to the physical organ that we know lies in the chest cavity to pump blood throughout the body. They were reporting a primal experience that we share today.

In negative situations there is an almost instantaneous constriction or hardening there. In positive experiences, there is an almost instantaneous expansion and softening there. Probably before the emotions were categorized, the experience of expansion or constriction registered. These reactions are not only spontaneous but pure—they cannot be manufactured. Selfish pleasures that hurt others or compromise integrity can feel good at some level, depending on one's level of maturity. But the heart cannot lie: it cannot soften and expand when something happens that is not life-enhancing. While we think of the ten commandments and the moral laws of other religions as imposed on us from a position of righteousness and obligation, it is possible that they actually arose from this most basic movement of the heart as it responds to various situations. Coveting, stealing, and the like may feed some of our basic impulses, but never result in that warm glow because they are not life-giving. And the divine intention is always to give and to affirm life.

Think of the metaphors language has to offer. We speak of the tenderhearted, the sweethearts, the ways we take things to heart or learn them by heart. People with true goodness are said to have hearts of gold. Those who cannot restrain their compassion are bleeding-heart liberals. A sincere thought is heartfelt, and a good story is heart-warming. By the same token, we don't want to get on the wrong side of those who are hard-hearted or cold-hearted or who have a cheating heart. All of these people are, in fact, deemed heartless, although we know very well that they do not lack the physical organ. They are damping the energy that could be flowing unimpeded through that area of the field that is their body. They are not vibrating clearly there. Songs, too, remind us of these analogies. It is not just, "Come into my arms," but "Come into my heart." We fall for someone "Heart and Soul" (never brain and abdomen, although presumably they are also involved in the process). Hearts ache or are broken. I can ask you to open your heart or I can try to win it.

These do not refer to the physical organ per se. Of course, the organ itself is an important conduit. The medical establishment is now trying to come to terms with the fact that some recipients of heart transplants carry the memories and habits of those from whom they anonymously received this gift of life. How else to explain the sudden craving for chicken nuggets and beer experienced by a convinced vegetarian whose donation was from a young male who considered this party food? And scientists are studying the electromagnetic field around this area of the body to show that measurable waves have an impact on people's immune system and on the immune system of the other folks they interact with. I read clinical reports on this subject with wonder. They often corroborate what I intuitively know. But I am not a scientist, and I will leave this data to the experts, just as I will leave the task of uncovering the biochemical components of happiness and depression to others.

I am sharing here the attitudes and practices that have helped me live with a happy heart, recognizing that these attitudes and practices have been taught by many of the great spiritual traditions. I am concerned with fourth chakra energy, which processes the ability to be in warm relationship with oneself and others. Imbalance here makes itself known in various ways, many of them immeasurable. You may notice that there is an imbalance when grief does not subside over time and takes up permanent residence. Or you may be bitter about things that happened in the past and resent the circumstances that brought you to this point. These are signs of deficiency. There can also be excess. You may classify yourself as co-dependent or simply notice that you get very clingy when you love. Perhaps you take care of everyone around you in the hope that they will stay near. All of these scenarios show an energetic imbalance. Love is not about pushing others away or hanging on to them. It is a dance between equals.

As we strive for balance, we also take note of the health of the physical organs around the heart. Here we come up against the idea of blaming ourselves for illness. If I am suffering from heart disease, bronchial pneumonia, or breast cancer, does taking heart chakra activity into account mean that I could have brought the disease on myself? Some people resist looking at the energetics of the situation for this reason. I asked one woman who had been trying desperately to conceive a child whether she had considered augmenting medical treatment with alternatives. "Oh no," she said, "I'd have to admit that I could have done something about this a long time ago and didn't." What a bind to be in! We are all capable of delaying the possibility of a longed-for outcome because we don't want to risk any guilt for choices made in the past. But blaming yourself for past decisions is not the issue. Let's start with the here-and-now.

You are responsible for what you are conscious of. You did not consciously create your problem. However, your problem can be a wake-up call. When Jesus traveled the countryside and met many sick people, He would usually ask, "Do you want to be healed?" We have no record of the ones who refused, although there were probably lots of them. No matter how appealing a new idea may be, my first impulse is often to ignore, refuse, or disbelieve it. Any important change in attitude or behavior, small or large, causes a major disruption to the whole system that is my life. So a problem in my physical, psychological, or social makeup may be my chance to look at an area of resistance.

When that happens, I do not blame myself for the glitch. That would be useless. What is useful is to take responsibility for assisting the healing process. If healing can be served by a revision of attitude or behavior, will I refuse it? If Jesus walks up to me, asking if I want to be healed, will I respond with a resounding "Yes," or will I ask for a little healing today and maybe come back for the rest tomorrow? Or will I say that I would like the chance to prepare everyone at home for the big change? Or will I need time so that I can take out my scrapbooks so that I mourn my past and plan my future? Healing is always offered in the present moment. You can resolve your heart disease—physical, emotional, or spiritual—by any means you choose. Just know that in every here and now you are deciding whether to accept or reject well-being.

Many of us are unfamiliar with the way the heart works. Think of it as the internal harmonizer. We can react from our gut feelings or we can be glued to the floor (stuck in the lower chakras), or we can weigh every move or float above our own lives (stuck in the upper chakras). People usually come down hard on one side or the other, although it is possible in the same lifetime and even on the same day to veer wildly between the two poles. Rare are the moments of clarity when we can acknowledge our feelings, bring reason to bear, find our inspiration, and choose the course. In these rare moments, we are neither totally impulsive nor analytically detached. We are present. We are coming from the heart.

"Not detached?" you may ask. "Don't most spiritual traditions teach detachment?" I used to ask that question myself. I disliked the sound of the word detachment and couldn't figure out if it was required in order to be spiritual. It conjures up the image of a person who is calm, cool, and collected. Or of one who is sterile, dispassionate, or neutral (in the sense of being neutered). I think that non-attachment is a better term to describe what the traditions teach. Practicing non-attachment means acknowledging feelings as they arise without hanging on to them. One woman in a workshop I was leading asked tearfully, "Am I supposed to smile and wave goodbye to my husband when he leaves me for another woman?" I hurried to assure her that a spiritual outlook is not cavalier or reckless. With a spiritual outlook, she will still be affected by people and events, but her feelings will not run her life.

To be in the heart is to practice non-attachment to the results of your own actions. Of course, you can still act with enthusiasm and enjoy the fruits of your labors, but you can't decide ahead of time what those fruits will be. As the old adage says, "Don't count your chickens before they're hatched." Before my own two wonderful chicks, a girl and a boy ten years apart, were hatched, I imagined all sorts of futures for them and for us together. I pictured my daughter in velvet and ruffles and my son in a little shirt and tie. Of course, Amy chose to wear a black knit shirt with neon accents during most of the second grade, and Seth was born with an aversion to any piece of clothing with buttons. How futile it would have been to have tried to remake them. What a waste of my energy and theirs. Yet many parents try to do just that with their children. And many husbands and wives try to do just that with each other. And most of us who have any ambition at all try to do just that with our own lives. It is not so much that the ambition itself is a mistake—the attitude with which it is carried out can be.

It is good to want to make something happen. It is fine to have a goal. But that something or that goal can look very different as events take shape. Since all of life is change, you want to be dedicated to your process without being fixated on a particular goal.

Love is what allows us to remain committed to the process of creation, and at the same time to drop our attachment to the outcome. Yet that is not the common wisdom about love. We think love means possessing a person or an idea. Held tightly, the possession can be shaped into the ideal, the plan can be turned into the product. But that is really obsession, not love.

When the heart is truly open there is no place for obsession. We seek only the best outcome, whatever that is. You can work passionately for a particular result, then temper the striving with the thought, "May all occur for my highest good and for the highest good of all who will be affected." This is because no one of us alone has the whole picture. What you think you want so passionately now may not serve you later on. You know the old saying: "Be careful what you pray for—you may very well get it!" Love is what keeps us unattached to the superficial and in touch with the soul's truest desires. It is possible to be peaceful and passionate at the same time. In fact, that is the soul's joy.

Many contemporary spiritual writers remind us to check in regularly with our feelings because the soul, our essence, speaks through emotion. This is true. When you are offered the new job that is everything you've been preparing for and are inexplicably enveloped in a cloud of sadness at the prospect of accepting it, you would be wise to re-examine your future plans. If the thought of moving from your fashionable four-bedroom home to a cottage on someone else's estate makes you happy, you would be wise to pay attention to the message. However, it is not sufficient to consult feelings alone when choosing a course of action. Feelings-in-the-raw can arise from chakras one through three. They are immediate and powerful sources of information, to be sure. But just as information from the upper regions must be processed through the center, so must those from the lower regions. You do not want to analyze or waft your way through life, as you would if you were to take direction from chakras five, six, or seven only. Neither do you want to find yourself gripped in the clutches of chakras one, two, or three. For instance, rage can live there. Of course, you want to acknowledge and feel rage as a valid emotion. It is telling you something about yourself, but until you sit with it and allow your heart space to receive it, you have no way of knowing whether this is anger over a perceived injustice or just the ego's first reaction against being thwarted. And you certainly cannot make a wise choice quickly about how to respond.

The heart takes a base emotional response and transmutes it into usable energy. This energy will still have the quality of a feeling, but it will be a feeling unattached to a particular action or outcome. For instance, the rage in chakra three, at the solar plexus, wants to kill. In chakra four at the heart, we can be open to the severe sadness or disappointment that has fueled the rage. We can comprehend from an expanded perspective that killing the cause of this sadness or disappointment does nothing to change the situation, which still cries out for healing.

But it is not just the obviously destructive emotions that require transmutation. Not everything we call love is heartfelt. Melancholy, sentimentality, clinginess, and jealousy can all be mistaken for love. But they originate in the insecurity that indicates a lower chakra deficiency or excess. Only when they are transformed in the heart is there true love. For instance, a feeling of jealousy that wants to keep another close by is what many mistake for love. But true love, while able to voice its desire for the beloved to stay, is finally able to sadly but graciously step aside when that is not the other's choice. True love may even be capable of wishing the other well, despite its own pain and suffering. Love is always its own reward, and any other benefits are a pure gift. Love purifies your vibration, and you and all you touch will reap its harvest of well-being. So graciousness in the face of disappointment is more about you than about the one who has wronged you. This is why spiritual traditions teach us to love our neighbors and our enemies. True love is committed to process but unattached to outcome, even to an outcome that it strongly desires.

If you want to know more about your soul, or essential self, look into the window of your heart. Place your hand on the center of your chest, breathe deeply, and stay quiet. You can almost literally take your heart's temperature. Pay attention to the words or images that come up. Pay attention especially to any words or images that seem to imply that the heart is hard, frozen, bitter, raw, sad, isolated, unprotected, armored, or the like. Instead of making excuses, just let yourself experience what's going on. Cry, speak, write, or scream about it. This is the start of healing. It can continue in any number of ways.

This is where you may want to enter psychotherapy. Psychotherapy is like going into each of the three lower and the three upper chakras to excavate the origins and status of each imbalance that can be named as a symptom. That is helpful, as long as you don't get stuck in your story — that is the opposite of the non-attachment that signifies the soul's health. Just as you don't want to be attached to a future goal, so you don't want to be attached to the past.

It is possible to understand yourself fairly well at the level of your wounds and never move beyond that. When your wounds identify you and provide a common ground for connecting with others, there is little impetus to heal. People who like to think of themselves as wounded may initially look intriguing, but don't seem very deep as you get to know them better. I once saw for a few times a young woman who had been in psychotherapy for years. When I asked her for her therapist's prognosis, she told me as a matter of fact that it would take at least a decade of weekly or more frequent sessions before she could hope to be even minimally functional on an emotional level. She was an attractive, highly placed executive who was interested in spiritual things. She could give me minute details of her childhood. Her main complaint seemed to be that her mother and father had held her to the strict and sometimes harsh standards of their immigrant culture. It was clear that she was not ready to move beyond her pain any time soon. She would not even entertain thoughts that there could be similarities between her experience and that of other grown children from dysfunctional families, much less acknowledge that there were perhaps others who had suffered worse abuse. Her world view was based on the fact that she had had the worst childhood imaginable. Her miracle in life was that, as her therapist kept assuring her, she had managed to survive this long.

If you want more wonder, more joy, more empathy than that in your life, don't stop with psychotherapy. Allow yourself to make friends with your soul by getting to know the needs of your heart. Familiarize yourself with how it feels when it's happy and how it feels when it's not. When you do, your spiritual center of gravity shifts, and you become attuned to a higher frequency. A variety of teachings, tools, and techniques are offered in the following pages. Pick and choose among them and allow your rainbow to emerge.

CHAPTER 3

EMBODYING LOVE WITH YOGA, BODY AWARENESS, AND ENERGY BALANCING

I first became aware of my heart chakra when I was in a yoga posture. Until then, I had taken no notice of its presence. I assumed the physical organ must be in there because I was still alive. But the heart as a center of energy was nothing but a nice theory. Love itself remained a philosophical theory for me. Of course, I had had some experiences of love, most notably at the births of my two children. I remember bonding with my daughter when she was about three weeks old, lying on the doctor's examining table. I could see her vulnerability and felt a softening in the center of my chest. I did not recognize it as the movement of a new energy within me and, indeed, did not associate it with my heart at all. If I had, I might have used it as a barometer for deciding when it was safe to open myself to others in my life. I could also have anchored the emotional feeling of love with the actual tactile feeling in my chest. But I was disengaged from my body then, so I continued to protect myself, even with my daughter in her first few years. I just didn't know any better. It was easier to think my way through motherhood than to feel my way. Much as I loved Amy, I was still attached to previous occurrences in my life that made it dangerous for anyone to come close to me. I often experienced her little demands as big intrusions. Luckily my transformation began as she got older. My son who was born ten years later has fared better than Amy. I was a different person by then.

Soon after Seth's birth, life hurt too much and stress was taking its toll on my body. I picked up every illness the kids had, almost in triplicate. So I began to experiment with the connection of body, mind, emotion, and spirit, fueled by books and local workshops. I was still a parish pastor and had to do this other work quietly, given the suspicion of all things smacking even remotely of the "new age" common to many mainstream congregations. I began to eat more natural foods. I also began to meditate regularly and incorporate exercise into my life in a way that was also meditative. Soon I realized I needed to begin to study yoga again. My body became more fit, my mind more flexible, my emotions more available, and my spirit more connected with everything good.

The word yoga means yoking or union. You can picture this union happening vertically, connecting you with ultimate reality, and also happening horizontally, gathering the various parts of yourself—body, mind, emotions, and spirit—into a working whole. Yoga is a set of practices aimed at helping you to do all of this. Students regularly come into one of my yoga classes asking if we're about to do hatha yoga. I explain that all yoga that uses physical postures is hatha yoga. Hatha is merely a combination of the words for sun and moon in Sanskrit, so again we get the sense of opposites joining for a purpose. Within hatha yoga, there are lots of styles that have been handed down through various schools. This is not a yoga manual, but I will describe briefly some of the typical postures that will help your heart energy. If you are new to this, pick up a book or a video for beginners, or better yet, find a weekly class. If you are unfamiliar with what's available, try a few teachers and assess their style, training, and competency. Then choose a teacher and consent to let her or him guide the hour-long session. This letting go is a big step in the right direction. A good yoga class feels wonderful and over time will change your body. But please realize that yoga was never intended to be a cosmetic or quick fix. It was intended as a way to deepen consciousness.

Yoga originated in ancient India before writing was common, so it comes to us from the mists of history as part of the mixed bag of meditative practices from great spiritual teachers. Postures were not even part of yoga in the early centuries. Somewhere between 200 B.C.E. and 200 C.E. these meditative practices were printed in the Yoga Sutra. Posture was mentioned there only as a means of sitting still so that the mind can get clear. Later masters found that more elaborate postures, done with total attention to their complexity, could facilitate awareness. So they developed specific poses and countless variations that imitate natural objects such as plants and animals. Handed down to us, these postures work on many levels at once. On a physical level, they tone the body, strengthen the muscles, and massage the organs. On an emotional level, they invite you to feel the nuances of each stretch and to register how that stretch triggers a response such as fear or anger. On a spiritual level, the intensity of the physical moves can make you concentrate on the space that happens between thoughts rather than on your own inner chatter. And you will become aware of a dimension of human experience that is beyond doing and thinking.

There is also an energetic level to yoga. What fascinates me is the way each position activates our ability to embody similar energy of plant, animal, or whatever else it imitates. When you do tree pose, for instance, you reach high into the air with the spine and extended arms while balancing on one strong, root-like leg. You embody everything positive about tree-ness: how a tree can stand for years drawing its nourishment upward through its roots even in dry soil; how it reaches down into the ground as far as it must in order to get what it needs, and at the same time reaches tall into the sky in order to find any possible ray of sunlight in the densest forest—how it is grounded and lifted at the same time, deeply rooted, yet leafy and open to possibility. To do this posture is to embody both the tenacity and the flexibility that can live together in one physical form, indeed, that must live together if the tree is going to stay alive and healthy.

Every posture is a seed, in that it embodies an energetic principle. Because yoga is as concerned with awareness as it is with body positioning, that energy becomes even more available when you are focused than when you move in a similar way while thinking of a hundred other things. Attention is brought to the places where change is possible, and so change begins to happen.

Breathing helps the process. Check your breathing right now. You're probably breathing very lightly through your mouth and nostrils. Air comes down no lower than your throat or upper chest before you let out a quick exhale. Your attention is everywhere but on your breathing, which means that your attention is everywhere but on this moment. However, this moment is where your life is taking place. Why would you want to miss it? Besides, it takes much more effort to ignore what's going on than to deal with it. So use your breath.

Breathing is the only thing you must do now. You cannot use your breath from yesterday and you cannot store it up for tomorrow. If you aren't breathing right now, you are not alive in your body. When we die, it is said that we expire. When we live, it is to inspire. This, according to the dictionary, means to inhale, to animate the mind or emotions, to stimulate and influence, and to elicit or create. Inspiration is the universal creative energy, and it begins for us with our first breath. The word for breath, air, and spirit (life force/energy) is *prana* in India, *chi* in Asia, *pneuma* in Christian Greek, and *ruach* in Hebrew. It is telling that one word in each tradition has all these meanings. When we breathe deeply, we attune ourselves to divine vitality. It is more than just physical. In fact, even when we are physically or mentally ill, there is a place in us, accessible through the breath, where we are well. This well-being is felt in the heart.

So sit comfortably on the floor, either cross-legged, if you can sit that way without moving much for a while, or on a chair with your feet planted on the floor, your back not slouching into the chair. Pull your hands back onto each thigh, or lay them on top of each other by your abdomen. This pulls the shoulders back and opens the chest. Let your shoulders and all the tension they carry drop down, away from your ears as your spine loosens and lifts. Take your breath in through the nose, draw it down into the throat, then into the heart, then into the abdomen. Chest and belly become like inflated balloons. As the air floats downward, let it expand into your sides. Savor for a moment the feeling of being fully oxygenated. Then pull in the navel and let the air move up—out of your belly, out of your chest, through the throat and out the nose again. The balloons deflate. Savor this moment also. Choose to inhabit fully that moment of trust when all air is gone before taking the next breath. Allow your consciousness to follow the path of breath in and out, down and up, over and over again. When thoughts from the inside or distractions from the outside come up as they will, gently bring yourself back to the path of breath. Thoughts and distractions are like dots in a children's puzzle. You do not have to connect the dots into a complete picture. You merely notice that the dots appear and let them drift away. Many people tell me they aren't good at meditation because they keep being distracted. I reassure them that the Buddha didn't become the Buddha (the Enlightened One) after only a few meditation sessions. So don't feel bad or blame yourself because the dots appear. They will continue to be there as long as you're human. Meditation is the process of noticing and letting go of them. It is not the goal, but the journey. If you're on the journey, you are good at meditation.

This is the kind of breathing you will do during yoga poses in order to let their seed energy enhance your way of being in the world. It allows you to be fully present and therefore perfectly attuned to what the posture has to offer. You do not think about what is going on in your body; you become what is going on in your body. That subtle shift in emphasis makes a revolutionary difference because it takes you out of your head. It's probably more correct to say that it allows your head to be just one small part of a total experience. But how does this happen? Breathing deeply and completely, you move your awareness out of your brain and into whatever area of the body is being affected. Consider the brain to be the computer that organizes the data of your life. The data itself can be experienced firsthand as it emerges from every cell. However, it is often censored by the brain as it seeks to protect you from pain. Wisdom happens when you allow yourself to access the primary data before it is filtered through the distortions that have been created in the brain as reactions to prior experience. In chakra talk, you are then a flow of energy unimpeded by fear-based thoughts.

The posture in which I first experienced my heart chakra opening was a supported fish, a pose done lying on your back with your hands at your sides. You raise the mid- and upper back from the floor with the help of a rolled blanket or small pillow placed just under the shoulder blades. This allows the chest to lift and the head to tilt backward. The larger the blanket or pillow, the higher the chest rises and expands. There came a time when my body craved this posture and I wanted a substantial blanket or pillow underneath me while I meditated for perhaps twenty minutes to a half-hour at a time. The surprise for me was that I would sometimes begin to cry while in the pose. I was not unhappy about anything specific, certainly no more so than before I got down on the floor. It was my first inkling that moving my body could have such a strong effect. Certainly I had realized before that certain ways of moving could help me feel better or worse. For instance, I knew that dancing could make me feel great, even when I was not feeling that great to start with. But this was different. It was not about how the pose made me feel. I did not feel better or worse in supported fish. Emotions were tapped that had nothing to do with my subjective feelings. I could cry without being particularly sad or joyous, because it was the underlying energy that was being released. And my heart was the place it had been stored. Like a crumbling dam, my body at the heart center served to encourage rather than to impede the current. I literally felt my heart soften during these sessions, and there was a warmth that was unfamiliar. I had perhaps experienced it before, but always fleetingly, never in such a concentrated and prolonged state and so identified with one particular part of my body. I knew something important was happening, but I could not have predicted then how it would change my life.

The poses you'll want to do in order to actively stimulate the heart chakra involve opening, lifting, and expanding the front of the body. These can be warrior-type postures that involve standing with your hands placed together as in prayer at the center of the chest and then opening or lifting the arms. You breathe into the wideness of the shoulders and chest cavity that is created by the open arms. The same effect can be created in back bends such as locust or cobra where you lie on the abdomen and let the inhale carry your head and chest up several inches. As you draw your shoulders down and back, there is a bending of the spine but also a forward movement of the chest. Camel is another wonderful example. You can get the same effect by sitting on the floor with your legs in front of you, resting your hands on the floor by your hips. Using your inhale, you tip your head back, draw your shoulders back, and press the chest forward and up. The important thing is to make use of any posture where you expand the front of the body and keep your attention there. Contrast the effects of the lifting and backbending portions of your practice with those of the folding and forward-bending portions. Of course, any good practice will incorporate both of these types of movement for counterpoise and balance. Even if you decide to devote a half-hour session to postures that lift and open the chest with the intention of tapping into hidden heart energy, you will still want to intersperse and close with, for instance, some hanging forward bends and child's pose. Otherwise, your body will be unbalanced and your vitality somewhat frenetic. Besides, the symbolism of the heart opening is best expressed in the softer poses of surrender, and you will probably find yourself desiring them.

Of course, you can only spend so much time on the yoga mat. And you may choose never to enroll in a class or to develop your own practice. But that's okay. Practice is just that—practice for real life, for moving, breathing, deciding, acting. Your mat is a good lab, but it is only that. Whatever you do in a posture, you will also do during the day. If you hunch, tighten, clench, deny, over- or under-use parts of your body as you do yoga, you can probably find yourself doing the same thing sitting at your desk or waiting to do your banking. If your mind wanders unchecked, straying into reverie or planning; if it constantly makes comparisons and judgments; if it readily assigns or accepts blame; if you are easily bored, frustrated, anxious, or angry, you will typically find these attitudes creeping in as you talk on the phone or drive your car. Of course, we all have these tendencies because we are human. They do not go away on their own, but their impact dissipates when we notice what is going on and choose to let go, allowing energy to flow freely once again.

As a yoga teacher, I often guide students to become aware of their habitual attitudes of body or mind. We all do have all of them from time to time, but most of us have just one or two that predominate when we leave the moment. So I must regularly remind one student to keep her toes on the ground in standing postures and another to loosen her fingers when hanging in a forward bend. One young man never notices that his shoulders are clamped by his ears in seated forward bends. Others practically have smoke coming out of their ears from the mental energy they are burning in order to strive, compare, and berate themselves. These are not just once-a-week habits. They reflect something basic about the ways in which these people get in their own way whenever they lose awareness of the present.

You will lose it sometimes. What's important is that you get it back. How you do this is up to you. You can do "unofficial" yoga by building awareness into your aerobics class or weight training. Really be present to what's happening in mind and body instead of letting your attention wander. Yoga can be as creative as a headstand or as simple as becoming conscious of the way you walk. For instance, we all have a natural center of gravity, but often our minds have misplaced it. Try walking across the room with your center of gravity between the solar plexus and the heart. You move with grace and assurance, your top and bottom halves well anchored and working in tandem. But not everyone you see on the street walks that way, as you'll notice if you do any people watching at all. Try walking across the room with your center of gravity in your left hip, as it might be if you were favoring it because of a physical injury. What if you lead with your pelvis, as if your sexuality were your calling card, or with your head, as if you've got to figure it out before you get there? I was told by a chiropractor that conscientious counselors and therapists tend to have lots of neck and shoulder problems because they are always listening to others and trying to let the others see that they are listening. The only way they know how to do this active listening is to thrust forward their necks and cock their heads. Experiment with listening from your heart instead. Your neck and head can stay very relaxed while your chest radiates acceptance. It will make a difference to the way you feel and it will have a subliminally relaxing affect on the person sitting across from you.

Everyday actions have the power to facilitate or to diminish well-being for yourself and others. They can demonstrate how easily life happens or how tough it is. You can embody love just by walking from your true center of gravity, dropping and widening your shoulders, and becoming aware of the heart chakra's warmth so that you can project it out into the world. Do so, and you will become a blessing to all those you pass on the street. Positive energy affects in like manner all the other energy fields it meets, as does negative. A blessing is an attunement with what is life-enhancing and therefore sacred, combined with an intention to be a reminder of that attunement. Once you feel superior, you have lost it. The intention can only be borne from the realization that all other beings also carry with them the ability to be attuned with you.

If you have never done this, try a one-day experiment. Go about town to accomplish your errands as if your heart chakra were completely open and whirling. Feel warmth move between your solar plexus and your chest. Let that warmth radiate outward to others. Let it also radiate upward into relaxed shoulders and jaws and a soft face that smiles easily. How does the daily routine feel to you now? How do people respond? How does that feed your inner light? Life becomes, not a vicious circle of lament and loss, but an empowering circle of gratitude and riches.

It will be easier to find your heart space on sunny days when things are going your way, but you will need to be able to find it on rainy days when you have just suffered a disappointment. Approach the sunny days as if you were in training for, indeed, you are. After all, it often seems easier to locate and bemoan the one cloud than to celebrate the sun. So familiarize yourself with the way your heart feels when it is happy. Put your hand on your chest, breathe deeply, and picture some being (another adult, a baby, someone who has already left the body, a dear pet, even someone you can only imagine) whom you love without judgment. How does the area around your chest feel? Remember that the chakras do not merely affect one half of the body but permeate it. Experience your heart as it radiates into your back and feel its energy vibrating there. Register the physical and emotional changes that occur during such an encounter. Notice how you would describe life at this moment. Then, keeping your hand there and continuing to breathe deeply, again picture a being, perhaps not the same one, who has that kind of unconditional love for you. How does it feel to bask in such acceptance? Notice how it feels not to have to protect yourself. Perhaps after you have done this exercise enough, you will not even need to remember the particular beings consciously. Just placing your hand on your chest will trigger the experience of well-being and joy that is engendered by such unconditional love.

A simple gesture can create an opening in the vibrational field. The spiritual teacher Bhagavan Das advised me to take my index and middle finger together and tap a small circle at the center of my chest if I was feeling a little down. Mitchell May, a shamanic healer who allowed his own nerves and shattered bones to mend from what the medical community twenty-five years ago deemed irreparable damage, suggested larger movements. "Dance, stomp, and wriggle to world-beat or rock music. Don't worry about what you look like or about aligning the chakras. Just keep moving the energy upward from the lower chakras where it pools. That in itself is a big step toward healing." Now instead of sinking into mild depression or allowing myself to feel disconnected from life, I move the energy physically and notice that there is a corresponding movement on a deeper level. A simple gesture or movement, and I find myself moved emotionally, but it doesn't stop there. What we are aiming for is not just a warm fuzzy, for only a fool could imagine that we can get to a place where life is always cozy. We tap into that well-being and joy that undergirds existence, whether right now that existence feels sad or happy, poor or rich. Your gut-level feelings will let you know what seems wrong with life, and your thoughts will prod you to seek a remedy. Your heart, as the soul's window, will remind you of a joy that is pure buoyancy and remains constant through disappointment and fulfillment.

Given that your field is capable of renewing and adjusting itself, why might you call in a healer? Well, if our systems are like self-cleaning ovens, sometimes we want to invite someone in to turn on the heat. That is the effect such a person can have. Good healers will assure you that they are not the ones accomplishing the healing. (Let's not use the word "cure," for that implies merely the relief of symptoms. Sometimes the symptoms remain, but wellness is facilitated. Even when symptoms are relieved, the well-being achieved is much deeper than that.) Good healers will say they are merely conduits of an energy that flows through them. On some level that is not necessarily conscious, you give them access to your own imbalanced field so that your system can adjust itself. Anyone who takes credit for that is dangerously misguided, neither bowing to the ultimate source of his or her abilities nor empowering you to recognize that it is your own being that has invited, accepted, and made use of the process.

Whatever their specific gifts or training, true healers take over where your inner resources begin to sag. Keeping abreast of your own spiritual (read "total") health is a full-time job, because it demands consciousness, and consciousness is the task of a lifetime. But it is not a task you must or even should try to accomplish on your own. It is always a collaborative effort. This may seem strange at first. If I am responsible for my own attitude toward life, and I am, how can my enlightenment be a collaborative effort? Remember, though, that the world's spiritual traditions have always taught that a community effort is far more effective than an individual effort. People are encouraged to bond into groups so they can assist each other with physical needs and uphold one another in the spiritual quest. Contemporary research demonstrates that this interdependence is basic to the structure of reality. Life is a series of overlapping energy fields. It is revolutionary to look at each other as overlapping energy fields rather than as isolated individuals. We are swimming in a soup of energy, some of it denser (rock), some of it lighter (air), some of it balanced between the two (us). That is why studies are beginning to confirm that prayer works, whether it is offered by yourself for yourself or by others far away without your knowledge. Now many people are augmenting their medical treatment with methods of healing that only a decade or two ago might have seemed naive such as prayer, or odd such as reiki.

You may be baffled by the wide variety of choices available. There are methods that concentrate on nutritional and herbal remedies and those that use yoga and massage therapeutically. There are many types of healing touch. Reiki and acupuncture are standard offerings in the holistic marketplace today. Some people have devised their own repertoires of techniques. They go to Hawaii to study with a kahuna, to Africa to practice drumming medicine, to South America to apprentice as a shaman, to the American west to experience authentic sweat lodge. Each practitioner digests what has been learned, packages it, and offers it to the public. Are they all doing different things, or are they doing the same thing in different ways?

Again, the concept of vibration is the unifying thread that runs through the various styles of complementary medicine and preventative care. While it would be oversimplifying to say that they are all doing the same thing, it is important to understand that they are basically working with the human being as an energy field rather than as an enclosed system. The same way your own movements and attitudes are either expanding or contracting your flow, the people around you are either expanding or contracting your flow. Your practitioner will be a major influence on your health and so must be chosen with care. Whether you are dealing with a major illness or with its prevention, you will need to call in a healer when you sense that some assistance is needed. There are some fine ones as well as some con artists out there. So whom do you choose?

Of course, the first step is to see whether there are minimum standards for the type of care you are considering and then to decide whether a potential provider meets them. Vigilance in this area will be very important if a modality is physically intrusive, such as acupuncture, or if you are seeking treatment for a serious illness. But external qualifications can never be the only criteria. The relationship you will forge is paramount. No amount of training can compensate for an egocentric personality. No credential can take the place of rapport. In order to facilitate balance, this person will be touching your heart, even when the technique used doesn't involve physical touch. So it is important that you find yourself able to breathe easily in his or her presence. Then your analytical mind can relax and your impulsive nature can be soothed. Positive relationship is a strong opener of the heart chakra, and a positive relationship with a healer can be a prototype for all others. Find someone you implicitly trust, even as you continue to take responsibility for noticing and voicing any questions you may have along the way.

I have been blessed with a fairly strong physical constitution. Recently I had a small taste of the power of restorative energy work. This was with sound, specifically with the sound of the six-foot Australian horn called the didgeridoo. Carved from a hollowed-out eucalyptus tree, its voice is that of the deepest hum of the earth's core. I have friends who play this instrument at drumming circles, and it always stirs and comforts me at the same time. One weekend evening I'd planned to attend a small event featuring a didgeridoo master, but a busy schedule had left me vulnerable to a cold that was lurking just at the edge of my awareness. There was a tiredness behind my eyes, and I considered not going to this gathering. But I got in my car anyway, first swallowing my handful of herbs and vitamins. I remembered how much I'd looked forward to this and knew that I could always come right home afterward instead of driving on to the next meeting with friends I had on my calendar. It was a good decision. Not just a musician, but also an energy healer, this huge and kindly man treated us to his wonderful sounds. He then walked around our circle in order to direct his instrument at some place in each person that he sensed could benefit from attunement. As he came toward me, my intention was clear. "I am open to healing," I said over and over to myself as I adjusted my posture into open-heart mode— face and neck relaxed, spine lifted, and shoulders wide, creating a spaciousness in the chest. I knew he would direct his attention to the area between my chest and ears. As the didgeridoo sounded, I relaxed into pure peace. Later, as I was getting into the car, I realized that I could easily make it to the next event. I can't say that the cold had gone away. It was still there, but it wasn't part of me any more. The tiredness behind my eyes had moved beyond its capacity to debilitate me, and I watched it like a passing acquaintance.

It kept passing and never returned. That cold never did develop into even a sniffle.

Could I have allowed this same healing myself with enough prayer and focus? I'm convinced that I could have. But that's a theoretical statement of faith, because I did not then have what it takes to do that. My personality needed someone whose presence and technique I trusted in order to put me in contact with my own innate well-being. I am always whole in spirit, but his intervention helped me manifest that wholeness in the flesh. Cultivate the physical posture and meditative outlook that attune you with the vibration of the divine. But never be shy about inviting or accepting the help of someone whose integrity you can sense. The intention of life is for energy to flow. Even physical death does not betray this intention, for energy doesn't die. It is merely transformed when the body fails. Until then, accept well-being at every level and from whomever it is offered. There's no prize given for going it alone or for making life difficult. We are each a circle of energy, and we are each part of an extended circle of energy that includes all others. It is irrelevant whose hands facilitate the healing, whose body moves, whose attitude can hold onto the certainty of health. It will be me one moment and you the next. It is a shared heart that reveals the soul's potential.

MEDITATION PRACTICES FOR THE DEVOTIONALLY CHALLENGED

What could be more problematic to an intellectual than the idea of devotion? In graduate school I was surrounded by many people who studied and taught every variety of religious experience, but only a few people admitted that they ever had a religious experience. Rarer still were those who prayed or practiced a traditional religious faith. Of course, as academics we were keenly interested in the habits of the faithful, and in theory we professed to admire them, but in reality we were mildly condescending toward them. For the most part we were not atheistic or agnostic. We simply hypothesized the existence of the Sacred and researched it religiously, but didn't know how to relate to it religiously or even spiritually. Focused on the big picture, we often missed the trees for the forest, and knowing so much, we found it difficult to participate seriously in the practices of those people who did them routinely.

However, graduate school fit my agenda perfectly. I had not chosen it to become more religious or more spiritual. I had chosen it because I wanted to know more about religious traditions. Identifying myself with any one tradition at that point would have limited my options, and I needed to keep my options open. Although at bottom I longed for my studies to make an impact on my life, I didn't want to short-circuit the process. I do remember watching the few who were able to integrate religious fervor and academic rigor. For instance, a beloved, well-respected professor who was also a priest was known to have a personal relationship with Mary, mother of Jesus. There was also a graduate student who took us to visit his ashram and the Hindu temple where he worshipped. I didn't understand either of these men, but I did envy them.

Of course, it never entered my mind that knowledge was the tool I'd always used in relationships. Because my childhood had been so difficult, I learned to use my brains to keep one step ahead of danger in all the relationships I formed, and it made sense that I would skirt intimacy with divinity the same way I skirted intimacy with people. I studied those people—I didn't engage with them. I studied spirituality—I didn't engage with it.

I did venture into meditation because it could be justified as good psychology. Moreover, it was a common practice: many students at that time were meditating and flirting with the type of Buddhism that encourages an empty mind. It was relatively easy for me to practice clearing out my preconceptions about reality, and the silence was soothing. Still, the Buddhist monks had a sweet reverence which I couldn't identify with. Although proclaiming to believe in nothing, they seemed to have an almost personal relationship with something. Attractive as their demeanor was, I discouraged any hint of that in myself. I wasn't ready for their deep wisdom, mistaking it for spiritual naiveté.

Were you one of those people who avoided any hint of reverence or devotion in your own spiritual practice? Are you like that now? Does it work for you? It wasn't working for me, and it doesn't work for a lot of people. The eleventh step in the 12-Step recovery program advises the persons who want to change their lives to seek "conscious contact" with their Higher Power. The type of contact and the nature of the Higher Power are left for them to define.

Healthy devotion is not demanded or coerced, never approached as duty, and neither based on nor precluded by any philosophy. If you have left behind the religion of your childhood with its image of a God who floats above the clouds, you may think that devotion has no place in your life. But I know people just like you who include reverence in their spiritual life. I know those who practice devotion while insisting that there is only one reality and that every appearance of duality is illusory. These people are non-dualists who understand the value of surrender. Richard Miller is a well-known advaita (non-dualist) yogi and psychotherapist whose demeanor is one of true reverence. When I asked how he reconciled his philosophy with his practice, he replied simply, "It's not a question of devoting ourselves to one person, idea, or thing. It's about recognizing that our very nature is devotion itself." That makes perfect sense to me. It's my ego that experiences separation and longs for connection. At moments when alienation dissolves, it is appropriate for the part of me that expresses itself as ego to bow before the whole. This surrender is not related to literalism, fundamentalism, or cult-like activity. I am surrendering to what is not myself, or at least seems not to be myself, acknowledging that there is more to existence than meets the eye. Devotion flows from the heart that is softened by this awareness, but devotional rituals can themselves soften the heart. Stop analyzing. Be deliberately reverent toward what is least understandable and most valuable. Bow before mystery.

You can call what is not you God, soul, emptiness, or the true state of consciousness. The twentieth-century depth psychologist, Carl Jung, called it the Self, as opposed to the same word written with a lower case "s." One of these names will probably appeal to you more than the others, or perhaps you will devise your own. Then you can have interesting, sometimes rather heated, discussions with friends and colleagues who believe differently. That is the stuff of scholarly debate, and it can be fun. It can contribute to the human store of knowledge. Enjoy it, but don't let it keep you locked in your head, and don't let it seduce you from noticing the tug of your own longing. Celebrate such intellectual activity, but be aware of its limitations. It will never give you the ever-illusive, one true answer that will make your life meaningful and help you to live more easily in your own skin. And that's what everyone who sees me for guidance is seeking.

Once my heart chakra began to open, I really noticed the tug of my own longing for connection. And I began to relate that longing to traditional imagery that I had previously filed away as archaic. For instance, I was walking by a Roman Catholic church one sunny afternoon and passed before an outdoor shrine. There was Jesus, pointing to his heart on his chest with one hand and blessing me with the other. This was the same image of the Sacred Heart of Jesus that I had seen over and over again in my childhood in church and on the holy cards we used to keep in our missals and trade like baseball cards. The image was the same, but now it engendered a classic "aha" moment. Soon I was taking frequent walks past that niche, dragging anyone along who was even vaguely interested. "Isn't that amazing!" I would say. "Jesus is pointing to his heart chakra." It hit me that what I was beginning to feel so minimally was what he felt powerfully at his core. The statue was illustrating an energetic truth: that Jesus is called the Christ because he was able to participate fully in the vibration of divine love. In him there is no alienation. His heart beats with the same compassion that creates the universe. Few Protestants have been introduced to this image, and most of us raised as Catholics know only the tacky art that usually depicts it. Jesus' face is pale and pious, and his bleeding heart is ringed with thorns. It's not surprising that few progressive Catholics appreciate it today. One free-thinking nun who is a gifted energy healer said, "It's really not my style of spirituality." Untranslated, it can bring up all kinds of negative conditioning from the past.

The Sacred Heart imagery that we know today developed from the Christian mystical tradition. It was transmitted through a canonized saint of the Catholic Church, Margaret Mary Alacoque, in France in the seventeenth century. In deep contemplation, she was visited by Jesus, who showed her a fire burning at the center of his chest and said in essence, "This is my heart. It burns with compassion for all of humanity." Acutely aware then of her own failures, she asked him to take her heart and remove its selfishness. He reached for it and put it into the roaring flames of his own. There it was purified by love and returned to her chest as a little heart-shaped flame. After that, she knew a constant physical pain at that spot in her body and considered it a reminder of her relationship with the divine. Her insistence that this aspect of Christ be incorporated into her convent's worship eventually led to its acceptance in the larger Catholic world. Widespread practices such as taking communion on the first Friday of every month and the ritual enthronement of the Sacred Heart in observant Catholic homes developed from the visions of Margaret Mary.

While I was a pastor in a Presbyterian church several years ago, I was asked by a few brave souls to lead a seminar on the Christian mystics. Luckily I had my own resources, for the church library did not contain even one book on the subject. That shouldn't have surprised me. Many mainline Protestant churches avoid the topic for two reasons. First, in moving beyond rationality, mysticism can open the door to dangerous forces. Hence, the exaggerated left-brained orientation of some congregations becomes a judgmental and dangerous force of its own. Second, those mystics were not Protestants—they were all Roman Catholic.

But, of course, that isn't true. Many of the most-studied Christian mystics lived before the Reformation in the sixteenth century that divided the church into Protestant and Roman Catholic. Before that there was one body of Western Christendom, albeit with interesting regional differences. The church into which Francis of Assisi, Italy (twelfth century), and Julian of Norwich, England (fourteenth century), were born was not Protestant, but neither was it Roman Catholic. Catholicism later on redefined and reconstituted itself in order to differentiate its beliefs from the Reformation. The Christian mystics belong to all Christians, and mystics of every tradition belong to the world. They are gifted, able to experience essence directly. Though they were influenced by the cultures in which they received their experiences, they were never limited by those cultures. Perhaps this is why institutional religion has often managed to ignore their existence.

Margaret Mary did not come to her vision of the Sacred Heart in a vacuum. Although the directives from Christ to her community were most clear, other saints before her had also venerated Jesus' heart as the pivotal symbol of their faith. For instance, 300 years earlier, Catherine of Siena had experienced intimate conversations with Jesus. At one point, in the midst of a rapture in which her physical senses were suspended, she perceived herself giving him her heart. Instead of returning it, he replaced it with his own. Let's look at her description from an energetic perspective. Catherine's encounter is an extreme version of the awareness of unity that is part of any mysticism. If the Christ and the creator pulse with the same rhythm, would not the Christ and his disciple experience a similar kind of union? The symbol is the physical organ, but the reality is the vibration of compassion, owned by no one and shared by all who embrace it. It can flow through one being and into another. It is love made manifest—the theme found throughout the scriptures, embodied by saintly people, and encountered first hand by the mystics. Years later in 1968, another Christian mystic, Teilhard de Chardin, in *Science and Christ* would envision the psycho-spiritual evolution of humanity with the same metaphor: "It is in the form of a single heart that we must look for our picture of super-humankind, rather even than that of a single brain."

But the Christian world did not come to its awareness of divine love in a vacuum either. Its roots reach deeply into Judaism, for Jesus (Yeshua) lived and died an observant Jewish man. The Jewish mystical tradition is a rich one, and its evolution spanned thousands of years. Like the yogic tradition, what was eventually written was the product of generations of unwritten knowledge and practice. The Hebrew scriptures themselves were committed to parchment only after becoming firmly fixed in the oral tradition of teaching and storytelling. They are full of what today's teachers often call multi-sensory imagery. They reflect an awareness that something more is going on beneath what seems to be going on; and so the sacred dimension is revealed. The "Song of Solomon," for instance, takes us into the world of two lovers and lets us glimpse in their statements to and about each other, not merely the intensity of their love, but also their ecstatic relationship with the ultimate source of their ardor. Human interaction reveals divinity at work.

In these scriptures, the whole process of divine guidance unfolds within the story of a persecuted people who never lost trust in God's overarching love and care even at the most difficult moments. God is sometimes ascribed characteristics we may find offensive, characteristics of the warrior or the judge. But we must take into account the ancient origin of these pieces and the consciousness that recorded them. In the Jewish tradition, these traits arise from the covenant made between the people and God, in which they were promised protection. Few scriptural references here or in the rest of the world's religious canon manage to note and empathize with the predicament of those others—the enemy—whom God is presumably also willing to protect and deliver. What is remarkable here is that, within its context, the Hebrew text continuously uses words for mercy, compassion, love, and loving-kindness to describe what it knows of God. It is this understanding that nurtured the

Jesus whom Christians follow. It is what prompted the flowering of mysticism in both Christianity and Judaism in the centuries following the end of the first millennium C.E.

In the years between the twelfth and seventeenth centuries mysticism flowered in both cultures. We have seen the importance of the heart in Christianity then. In Judaism, much of the activity took place in Spain until in 1492 Isabella evicted everyone who would not convert to Christianity. Saint Teresa of Avila who lived in sixteenth-century Spain came from one of these "converted" Jewish families. One of her transrational moments is immortalized in the Bernini sculpture of an angel piercing her heart with an arrow.

The Zohar or Book of Radiance was written there somewhere after 1275. In many ways, this was a zenith in the movement we now know as Kabbalah, which literally means "tradition." Wordy, weighty, and of unclear authorship, it systematized knowledge that had become available over the previous thousand years in the rabbinical commentaries and in the spiritual lives of the devout. It also served to feed a mystical stream of Judaism that would bubble just below the surface and emerge in movements such as early eighteenth-century Hasidism and twentieth-century Jewish Renewal.

In the Kabbalah, there is first of all Ayn-Sof—Godself—mysterious and unknowable. That primordial consciousness creates relationship through its ten attributes, or *sefiroth*. These ten can be laid in a pattern to form the Tree of Life, indicating their interplay in the creation of the entire natural world. More relevant for our purposes is that they can be superimposed on the human form as the Adam, the earth being. Interestingly enough, although ten, they are arranged in ones and twos to embrace seven sites on the body, from lower spine to crown, reminding us of the seven chakras. This should not be too surprising once we understand the reality of this energetic information that shows up in various guises from culture to culture.

The sefiroth are living energies, ranging from shekinah at the bottom—the feminine indwelling presence—to keter—the supreme crown at which potential begins to actualize. In between are qualities such as wisdom, understanding, endurance, majesty, and righteousness. At the center of the body is the heart center. Today it is often called tiferet, which means beauty, although in other times it was more commonly called rahamim or compassion. Just above and to either side of it are the sefiroth of judgment/power on the left and mercy/kindness on the right. Tiferet's role is to mediate between the two sides, between judgment and mercy or between power and kindness, depending upon the emphasis. These pairs are not divisions but are intended to work together. True justice is not hesitant to name its recompense and consequently does not feel diminished at extending mercy. True recognition of one's own power results in a desire to affirm the power of others, hence the kindness. But they do not work together without the balancing energy of the heart center which is active compassion, the practice of feeling the experience at hand. This is recognized to be an inherent attribute of the Sacred. It is also a way for a human being to become aware of the sacred dimension of existence and to embody it. Again it is the vibration of the beating heart that facilitates creative expression. Balance in the center leads to harmony between the extremes. What arises is the beauty of human nature when it is attuned to divine vibration and the flow of energy is unimpeded.

Both mystical Judaism and mystical Christianity have allowed heart imagery to move the spiritual ideal of love from the realm of the generic and abstract into the personal and practical. It becomes possible then to invoke compassion without framing it as an ethical demand. For the mystic, the ten commandments exist more as statements of truth, than as harsh moral injunctions. In other words, we are invited to love because that is our basic energy. To vibrate at that frequency is to experience an undeniable attunement with the way the world works at its best and with our own optimum well-being. In making this point, each tradition uses a personified heart to elicit an immediate and emotional response that awakens in us the latent desire to love. In Judaism, heart energy is embodied in the "every (wo)man" and in Christianity in the "anointed man." The important thing in each case is that it is personified and becomes available by extension to any seeker. Heart chakra energy thereby becomes as accessible in these traditions as it is to the yogi. A related movement can be found in Buddhism.

Buddhism is unusual among the world religions because it does not begin with any idea of, or relationship to, the divine. In fact, it initially rejects the concept of divinity because its task is to negate the reality of all concepts. Buddhism is about the purification of consciousness in order to perceive reality accurately. The Buddha was a man who made it his mission to unearth the ways in which his own mental projections created the world as he saw it. He found that becoming attached to these projections meant immediate or eventual suffering, because things either were not what they seemed or were for a micromoment and then went on to change. Those people whose minds could not take in the nature of discrete, ever-changing elements were doomed to a lifetime, or many lifetimes, of clinging desperately to a vapor and being constantly disappointed when it evaporated in their hands. Having realized this after a long period of trial and error, he perfected a way of maintaining such awareness from moment to moment. This he taught as the "middle way" between austere self-denial and utter self-absorption. It involved a meditative practice to assist people in meeting each moment as it arose apart from the conceptual framework with which it would ordinarily be viewed. Labeling himself a teacher, the Buddha asked only for the discipleship of those who were committed to learning his way of processing reality in order to break the cycle of suffering and rebirth.

After his death, a strain of Buddhism called the Theravada retained this direct approach to enlightenment, It has an appealing simplicity. Although you are encouraged to be in community (the sangha) for support in following the Buddha as your dharma (path) unfolds, the process is primarily an individual one, and each person must earn his or her own enlightenment. Buddhism developed a variety of expressions as it traveled from India to places such as Tibet, Nepal, China, and Japan. The Mahayana (Great Vehicle) allowed for a broad interpretation of the initial teachings. Words like "thusness" and "suchness" began to be applied to the emptiness of each moment and eventually took on attributes and qualities of their own. From this, a pantheon of gods, goddesses, and other supernatural beings developed. Even the person of the Buddha began to have overtones of divinity, as images of him were painted, sculpted, and set in shrines. (One beautiful image shows a jewel embedded in the center of his chest, at his sacred heart and another in his forehead, at the site of his third eye.) This process testifies to our reluctance to deny the presence of the Sacred. With this renewed willingness to embrace the sacred dimension, the description of the one who sets out to attain enlightenment changed also. Where first there was the arhat, the individual meditator solely responsible for his or her own process, eventually there was the bodhisattva.

The essence of the bodhisattva is a great, loving heart that manifests in human form the archetypal heart. It is the bearer of *karuna*, compassionate love for all sentient beings.

Because of this compassion, bodhisattvas are not satisfied with attaining their own enlightenment. They do not cling to the blissful state of nirvana attained through meditation and good deeds. They continue to mingle with all of us who are caught in the cycle of birth and death, vowing to stay present and available until every last one of us awakens. What this means on a practical level is anybody's guess. Do they physically die? Do they forego a heavenly experience after death so they can remain available to earthly life through prayer? Do they choose to be reincarnated to work among us despite the fact that all their lessons have been learned? What is more important than the details is the intention expressed in their vow and the implication it has for those of us seeking to live from our heart chakras. In just a few hundred years, Buddhism changed from the desire to escape one's personal suffering to a deep longing to bring such relief to the entire world. A subtle shift allowed it to maintain its commitment to awareness while recognizing that discrete elements, even people, are related on a deeper level than we see. There is an understanding in the Mahayana of an energetic connection that allows us to influence each other. So the bodhisattva can dedicate the fruits of his or her meditations and good deeds toward the salvation of other beings without violating the integrity of the dharma. And, as in the other traditions we have explored, this understanding is personified in the one who is living from the intelligence-heart (bodhicitta) or the great compassionate heart (mahakarunacitta). The heart chakra makes itself known, and theory must bend to love.

Does theory bend to love in your own life? Most of us are more intent on being right than on being well and happy. Once you are tired of being right, you may be ready to try something different. One way is to have your spirituality become more relational. Perhaps that desire has been there for a long time, but you've been afraid to look at it. Like the traditions we've just explored, you can incubate such a desire for as long as it takes and express it in any way that feels right. You are wise to shy away from any approach that seems coercive or demanding. A way to start may be for you to notice times when your body wants to bow or make some gesture of deference in the course of your daily activity or during your yoga or meditation practice. Notice, too, when your mind wants to flow into gratitude as it recognizes goodness and beauty. Then allow yourself to give expression to these promptings without stopping to think why or for whom they are meant.

Intelligent people like to critique such impulses, but sometimes we can be too smart for our own comfort. Learn to turn off the inner critic when the stakes are relatively low. This will give you some practice in trusting your body's wisdom and your own intuition. Allow yourself the luxury of spontaneously twirling on the grass, bringing your hands together over your heart, lifting your face to the night sky, or voicing a few words of thanks to no one in particular.

These can become part of your personal set of rituals. Initially such rituals merely express your joy and wonder. When used often and well, however, they can be powerful enough to trigger these positive feelings.

At this point, you have taken the first small steps on the path of bhakti yoga. As I said earlier, the average yoga class is hatha, utilizing body and breath as meditative tools. Under the general umbrella of yoga, some people are drawn to raja, deep meditation, others to jnana yoga, intense study and knowledge, still others to karma yoga, work and service. Then there is the path of devotion, bhakti. Psychologists who study personality types have recognized that each of us probably move toward one or two of these ways of processing life. Our preferences for the ways in which we are or are not religious fit into this framework. It seems as if we are born thinkers, doers, internalizers, or lovers. My own tendency was to be a thinker, and I placed myself in that slot when I was asked to describe myself at a spirituality workshop a long time ago. However, as I grew and worked with people on their spiritual growth, it has become more and more clear to me that our goal should not be to name ourselves but to allow our personalities to encompass bits and pieces of what is at first unfamiliar. The element of devotion is certainly one that can enhance and soften any of the others, for it is the way of the heart.

There are many meditative techniques to awaken the energy of the heart. The Buddhist meditation of *metta* (loving kindness) begins as usual in the cross-legged sitting on the floor or feet-flat-on-the-floor seated position described on page 62. Breathe deeply according to the instructions given on that page. After a few minutes, begin. On the inhale of your breath, visualize yourself and say, either silently or aloud: "May I be safe and protected from harm." With the exhale, say, "May I be happy and peaceful." With the next inhale: "May I be strong and healthy of body." With the next exhale: "May I live with ease and well-being." These are variations of the traditional Buddhist blessings, but you can certainly create your own four-part phrases. Don't be judgmental about your performance and do feel free to start over if you lose your place. Repeat these for a few moments in order to sense your own fullness. Depending on your situation, you can repeat these as long as you wish. It is not recommended that you try to bless others with things you do not experience as true for yourself. Once you do feel comfortable allowing these intentions into your life, you may choose someone whom you have tremendous regard for, picture that person, and direct the phrases to her or him with your breath: "May you be safe and protected from harm, may you be happy and peaceful, may you be strong and healthy of body, may you live with ease and well-being." You can then, but only as you feel ready and maybe not within one meditation session, address the blessings to someone who is neutral in your life, neither loved, nor hated, such as your regular supermarket cashier. Eventually, you will be able to send a blessing to someone in your life toward whom you feel anger, animosity, or fear. But don't rush to this part of the blessing out of a sense of obligation. Move slowly, and at some point you will truly want to send loving kindness to all beings.

The Tibetans offer a similar process called *tonglen* (sending and taking). With the same easy yet relaxed posture as before, begin your deep breathing. At some point after your mind begins to feel open and still, let your inhale take in the experience of hot, dark, and heavy, and your exhale breathe out the experience of cool, bright, and light. Now identify the inhale with a real situation in your life that is painful, and identify the exhale with healing energy. You can gradually include all those who are suffering in ways similar to yours (for example, all over-worked single moms). Then, as you are ready, the taking in and sending can become larger and extend to others you know and love, to those who are difficult, and to those you see on the street and have a hard time understanding. The important thing is to be willing to take in their pain and equally willing to let go of it as you send healing. This establishes a bond between you and those with whom you might hesitate to get involved. It illustrates the difference between involvement and enmeshment. On the heart level, we are already involved with each other. If you are enmeshed with someone else, or preoccupied with your own pain, no healing is possible.

Both of these meditations can be done without any reference to a source outside of yourself and the others you are blessing. That makes it easy for those people who would find such a source an impediment, but want to cultivate the heart chakra energy without violating their own truth. If that is not an impediment for you, or if making the spontaneous gestures and doing the above meditations has dissolved some of your resistance, you may want to try the following Sufi meditation. Since Sufis are mystics from the Islamic tradition, which is strongly monotheistic, the point is union with God as the Beloved. Become still through posture and breath and imagine in the stillness there is love that surrounds you on all sides, and above and below. Recognize it as God's love and let yourself sink into it. Realizing that no part of you is outside of it, feel sheltered and secure as you breathe it in deeply. Present and serene, you can watch all thoughts as they arise and compassionately drown them in the sea of love in which you float. Indeed, because you are not outside of this sea, the distinctions between you, thoughts, and God blur. Everything merges with the Beloved. Your heart begins to open.

You live as a self-conscious being in a physical body. That means you wake up each morning to an awareness of your own fragility. Just getting out of bed can seem a risky activity in a world where injury is possible and death inevitable. You'd be living in a fool's paradise if you didn't acknowledge the reality of your physical vulnerability. But can you also acknowledge an even stronger reality just under the surface? This reality doesn't depend on your physical existence and doesn't need to be validated by intellectual theory. It is what undergirds every philosophy and theology. You can ignore it with a doom-and-gloom attitude that makes a litmus test of physical vulnerability and projects it into every aspect of life. Or you can live with absolute certainty that, despite appearances, you are always being cared for. By practicing some of these exercises and meditations, you can allow yourself to feel loved, which is the only way you will ever truly give love. The choice is yours.

If you're still a little nervous about this approach, perhaps you'd be more comfortable beginning with affirmations. They are simply statements that affirm positive thoughts. They are not addressed to anyone, but are read or said to oneself. If you haven't done this before, start with a fact that is true for you right now, one that you would like to keep in mind, although you know you might be tempted to forget it. It might be, "This is an interesting time in my life," or "I have a nice group of friends." The trick is to write down your affirmations and look at them, or say them repeatedly so that they become second nature. Sometimes your world will seem boring or lonely, and you'll want to remember that that is not your permanent situation. Once a negative is perceived, it's natural to spiral into self-pity. It's easy to forget that the positive is just as true. And, of course, it is true on even deeper levels.

Once you've had the chance to use these basic affirmations, you can go deeper by noticing what you regularly say to yourself, especially when you contemplate doing or being more. We're always talking to ourselves, except that we tend to talk in negatives rather than in affirmatives.

Because the negations reveal our core beliefs, we need to examine them before discarding them. For instance, a thought might cross your mind that you'd like to apply for a different job or write a magazine article, or get out more socially. "Nah," you might find yourself thinking, "I'm just dreaming. I'd never be able to do that. Who'd want me? I'm safer staying where I am." This reveals what you believe about yourself as well as of what you believe about the world. The more inhospitable you perceive it to be, and the more you describe yourself as lacking what it values, the likelier it is that you will continue to feel shortchanged and, indeed, that will reflect the truth. The world cannot value what you do not. In that sense, you create your own reality, one in which it is unsafe to open your heart.

So make it a habit to notice the statements about yourself or the world in general that are passing through your mind. Choose one or two negatives that you notice fairly regularly and reframe them in a positive light. State them in a way that you can believe at some level, even though that may mean a stretch. You don't want to be so unrealistic that your statement feels like a flight of fancy, but you do want to move out of your customary comfort zone. For instance, it might be too big a jump for you to say and mean, "I am the company's next vice-president," It might not be a big jump to say and mean, "I am a talented manager of people." Again, write down your affirmations, tack them up where you're likely to see them, and repeat them often so that they filter into your consciousness and become your new reality.

They should be simple yet descriptive. "I am" is always a great beginning. Do presuppose that the activity described is already completed. When you are making the heart a priority, there are plenty of ways to let in the assurances that you never before received or were offered but refused to believe. I have used, "I am receiving now all the love the universe has for me," and "I am surrounded by love and support as I offer my gifts to the world."

Imagery works in a similar way. Just as words are constantly popping up in your mind, so are pictures, and many are negative. Instead of picturing yourself accomplishing your goal, you picture yourself failing. Instead of imagining yourself surrounded by friends when you go to a party, you see yourself standing alone on the fringes. These reveal core beliefs, also, and can be changed. Notice how many of your inner pictures reflect fear. Do create a few new ones to reflect your growing confidence. Build on positive experiences you have had, such as a teacher's smiling face as you got a math problem right (even if it was one of the few times that happened), or how it felt to land your first job or experience your first kiss. Transfer that pride to an event you would like to see happen and create an image for it, including scents, sounds, feelings, textures, even tastes. Substitute it for the image that creeps in whenever you dream of possibilities. Use the positive images whenever you daydream and allow them to fuel your activity. Then watch your imagination create a new reality.

Yes, reality does change as you make a habit of practicing these kinds of meditative exercises. All of the physical, mental, and emotional experiments in this book are designed to help you become more comfortable with what is and at the same time more open to what can be. But they do take work. A certain focus is needed. What if you're just not up to it? One of my clients was recounting a difficult week and a mild depression that had led him to his yoga mat but left him without motivation to do what he knew would work. "I was miserable," he reported, "I couldn't even meditate. What else could I have done?" "Well," I replied, "perhaps you could have tried praying." He looked at me with a mixture of incredulity and relief and said, "It actually crossed my mind that it's okay to pray, but I didn't want to seem foolish." That is the plight of today's sophisticated seeker, a plight that would make no sense to the peasants I met in the Italian Tyrol, for instance, who considered keeping up their roadside shrines as important as the planting of their vegetables. We deny ourselves the comfort that simpler folks take for granted. So my client and I discussed appropriate ways for him to call on a Higher Power in times of distress. For example, he liked the idea of asking for help in dissolving his resistance to the yoga and meditation that would help him.

Why have we who are spiritual seekers gotten to the point where we are ashamed to admit that we pray? After all, even scientists are now proclaiming in popular magazine articles that prayer works, which comes as no surprise to millions of us who belong to prayer chains and prayer circles around the world. Recalling our assertion in the last chapter that consciousness is a collaborative effort, we can be sure of one thing. We are never in this alone. At the very least, we are in this with each other. Remember that we are overlapping energy fields swimming in a sea of energy the very essence of which is love. Isolation is a point of view we impose on ourselves. As with the metta and tonglen meditations, prayer for ourselves or for others is healing, whether or not we see physical effects. "Okay," you may ask, "so there's me and there's you, and we're not as separate as we look. But who am I praying to?" Remember that heart imagery in the three major traditions we explored was used to acknowledge a relational quality within ultimate reality. You need not buy into a concept of the "old man in the sky." You merely need to be willing to recognize that the sea of energy in which you swim is more, not less, conscious than you are. Love is personal, and by definition, "it" (the pronouns are always problematic, for no he, she, or it suffices) is Love at the highest frequency. As Tillich said, Ultimate Reality can be personal without being a person.

How do you begin to relate to something whose very nature is pure love? First take it in with breath. Stay with silence for a while. Then think and say whatever comes to mind. This kind of Consciousness cannot be made angry by what you say or don't say. In fact, saying something is the first step. Just give voice, mentally or out loud, to any longing, gratitude, anger, worry—whatever's in your heart. You might wonder whom you're talking to. Are you talking to yourself? Maybe the answer is yes and no. Your essence, that place where you and the sacred meet, is love. Essence can infuse your personality, but it is not your personality. So, while you are intimately connected with the one whom you address, your ego cannot claim to be that. Allow yourself to speak personally to that level of reality that is more than your ego and deeper than any layer of the unconscious you have uncovered in therapy or meditation. You can call that reality by any name you wish. Just don't get sidetracked by the philosophical whys or wherefores. Essence is beyond all human categories, but you are human and must relate to it in your limited way. Here and now you live as one body among many. You're not stuck there, but you must take it as your starting point. Hindu thought considers this diversity to be the result of lila, which means divine play. The Judeo-Christian tradition says it stems from God's longing for relationship. In a sense, all of our relationships are play—experiments in knowing and being known and ultimately knowing oneself. In fact, our worst relationships happen when we try to fit them into a theoretical framework that is too tight. Look at the ways in which the baggage of marriage can overshadow the actual relationship between two people. Intimacy must have a component of playfulness. So allow yourself to be playfully intimate with what is most loving and what is, for the moment at least, "not you." Call this prayer.

Pray for yourself and others. Picture the person you pray for residing in the deepest chamber of your heart, and surround him or her with loving attention as you raise your intention. The intention can be as specific as you like, but it is always wise to temper it with the acknowledgment that healing can happen on unseen levels and with surrender to divine wisdom, which will accomplish all for the highest good of you and the other. Holding a person in your heart is an amazing way to go, for that very act creates a spaciousness in your center that unblocks the dam. Words may not even be necessary. Remember that every prayer you pray, like every thought you think, blesses or diminishes you as well. So you don't want to call down retribution on someone who has wronged you. Count on the laws of cause and effect to work. You are entitled to release your feelings about what happened with words, tears, or non-harmful actions and to acknowledge the reality of what and whom you have experienced. But you don't want to pray for anyone in a harsh, manipulative, or even a self-righteous way, for your vibration will be affected just as surely as the other person's by your negativity.

Why pray? Religions will give you commandments, and theologies will give you explanations. But I'll give you a more personal answer. Prayer is a way of staying in touch with what is absolutely and eternally good, true, and loving without the burden of having to describe yourself that way or of having to make yourself that way. It allows you to be human, vulnerable, and flawed. It lets you ask, vent, lament, thank, and praise what you need not understand. Paradoxically, in acknowledging your human frailty, you give yourself the chance to become strong. In acknowledging a deeper source of compassion, you activate your own heart chakra.

LOOKING FOR LOVE
IN ALL THE RIGHT PLACES

It's easy to look for love in the wrong places. Actually the very act of looking ensures that every place will be wrong. That's because seeking anything implies lack. And if you're lacking something as important as love, you've got to be feeling needy. And to the needy person, there's only insatiable hunger. Life seems to be either a desert where nothing edible grows, or a supermarket aisle filled with lush produce on a day when your wallet's back home on the dresser. It really doesn't matter if what you want is impossible to get, or if you don't have what it takes to get it. The hunger, the lack, feels the same. It feels terrible. A gaping hole opens inside, and you want to grab at whatever might fill it, even if it's not good for you.

In the name of romance, many of us have grasped at straws, deluding ourselves in the process. Sure, no experience is wasted; we learn even through our mistakes. But unless you're a masochist, what's the point? For you to make it a lifelong habit is to suffer needlessly. Why continually submit yourself to a punishment for a crime against the heart that is easily preventable? Of course, I use the word "easily" ironically, for rehabilitation involves seeing yourself with new eyes and changing your longings and their satisfaction in the light of the heart chakra. It is not easy to do, but it's very possible.

First of all, let's admit that all of us—married, single, celibate, rich, poor, male, female—long for love, and no matter how much we have, more is better. The ego never thinks it has enough. However, higher consciousness knows that enough is the true state. Hebrews praise God with the word *dayenu* (it is enough) after each of the ways in which God has manifested generosity. The process of naming each blessing and then calling it enough implies that any one of a multitude of blessings would have been sufficient in itself.

However, God's abundance is generous to the point of excess, which engenders wonder and rejoicing. But how many of us approach our lives with wonder and rejoicing? It's easy to overlook our bounty, especially when advertisers want us to be dissatisfied so that we can buy what is lacking from them. Statistics show that most of us think we'd be happy if we earned just a little more. It doesn't matter what our salary is—just a little more would make things a lot better. We have a similar attitude toward love. We see it as a commodity in short supply, partially because we are told that things we can buy will give us the edge in this market. But the scarcity model doesn't work. As soon as I imagine that there isn't enough love to go around, I imagine that I will be one of those people who never get their fill and thereby I generate a self-fulfilling prophecy.

You learned in the previous chapter what it means to be filled with love, and you now know what that feels like. You may be tempted to believe that the experience is an illusion and your hunger the reality. Know now that the truth is just the opposite. The moment of fullness, which is also the moment of emptiness, is the eternal now in which there is no longing. It is as real as it gets, as real as you can get. It is where you and ultimate reality touch.

Love is not missing from your life at all, for it is an energy that you carry with you always. What may be missing is a particular expression of love that you have not yet manifested. And, of course, the missing piece of the jigsaw puzzle is always the most important and seems the hardest to find. I counseled a couple who had loved each other before the fertility treatments they obsessively pursued in order to have a biological child. They had lost sight of what they did have as they tortured themselves and each other about what they didn't have. Meanwhile, a man with wonderful children bemoans the fact that he has not yet met his life partner. A woman with a wide circle of loving, supportive friends fixates on the family-from-hell in which she grew up. And the person who has created a stable nuclear family with spouse and children complains of having no best friend. Where does your dissatisfaction lie?

Let's begin by taking your heart's temperature. As we did on page 54, put your hand on your heart, breathe deeply,

and notice what comes up for you. If you feel negatives aris-
ing, notice what they are. Do not disregard your feelings,
but don't focus your attention there either. See if regular,
deep breathing brings you a measure of relaxation and fullness. Perhaps you will want to call up the experience of
unconditional love with the process described on pages
69–70. That can interrupt the vicious cycle that takes you
from need to longing, to loneliness, on to self-pity. Then
you can consider the particular expressions of love you do
have in your life. Do you have a good friend or two, a dyna-
mite kid, a loving partner, a sister or brother or parent you
can always call on to vent? Whether you do or not, let your
mind travel further afield. Acknowledge your congenial co-
workers, or the acquaintances who welcome you when you
meet at gatherings. Let your mind rest on distant cousins or
old friends who regularly keep in touch, even if only on hol-
idays. Think about the bank clerk who usually recognizes
you with a greeting. Count your pastor and your therapist
and your teachers or mentors at school and work. Don't forget your pets and friendly neighborhood animals. The point
is not to overlook any source of acceptance and support.
And that is exactly what we usually do. In our angst over
what we have decided isn't there, we forget to celebrate
what is there.

Please recognize the value of basic affirmations that
keep you in touch with what is. Feel free to construct a few
now based on the above information; for instance, "I feel
welcomed by _____ whenever I walk into

_____," "I can always call on _____ when I am feeling low," "I am blessed to have so many marvelous people in my life," etc., etc. Or create your own gratitude journal, promising yourself not to go to sleep at night until you've written down several things that happened during the day for which you are grateful. If you're praying more, as I suggested in the last chapter, you can incorporate thankfulness into evening or morning or anytime prayers. These are simple exercises that prepare you to invite the missing pieces of your personal jigsaw puzzle to appear.

Acknowledging what you have doesn't mean you can't also acknowledge what you don't. However, naming what is wrong with your life takes on a different quality once you have named what is right. Once you've done that, you realize that you're not starting from scratch. You have the outline of the puzzle. Now you need only check to see how far into the picture you've progressed. For some of you, the developing image will be very clear. For others, the scene will be fragmented and sparse. What matters is that something is there already, a framework on which to hang your life.

Why the missing pieces? Believe it or not, they are absent for a reason. They are useful—they can tell you how your mind works when it keeps you from realizing spirit's intention. The pieces that are in place cannot perform the same function, for they show how your mind has cooperated with spirit to bring about whatever is positive in your reality. Once you have what you've cooperated with spirit to attain, it's easy to forget how that happened. You don't remember the particular beliefs you held at the time which contributed to your success and paved the way for abundance. You've found a piece of your puzzle, and it seems as if things couldn't have happened any other way. I'll bet you're less complacent about the pieces that are still missing.

Let's look at this from the standpoint of your career. You may be unemployed or underemployed and indecisive about what to do next. For some unexplainable reason and despite your education and experience, meaningful work that pays well never seems to appear for you. That is a missing piece. Yet there may be a reason for this piece to be absent. For instance, a closer look may reveal that you have learned to live simply and not too shabbily on very little. That's a piece in place, probably a value that you wanted to manifest. Once you realize that and see simplicity as a lesson already learned, you will also realize that you don't have to learn it again. In other words, you don't need to be baffled by your career in order to stay close to your values. You can keep them and choose work that will support you on all levels. There'll be some effort involved, but you're probably already making it harder than it needs to be.

One of my clients struggled with this from the opposite perspective. A well-paid and respected corporate executive, she made money almost without thinking about it. She devoted herself to the company between nine and five and also did some business traveling, but basically she never had to work herself to the bone or give up her family life for success. She had the education and skills, and had obviously given herself permission to earn a fabulous salary. But when her artistic streak became more and more insistent at the onset of mid-life, she hesitated to even to begin preparing herself for a new career in design that drew her. The office was becoming less exciting every day, because the portion of herself that was engaged there was getting smaller. She really wanted to create beautiful environments for herself and others, perhaps even to the point of donating some of her work to people who would otherwise not be able to afford her. But she was afraid of losing her position and her money. What if she jumped from the frying pan into the fire and failed? At one point, I stopped the dialogue and asked her to look realistically at her monetary picture. What had she created in her financial life thus far? Once she saw that she consistently made responsible business decisions that allowed money to flow to her, she was able to admit that it was highly unlikely that she would now make a premature or downright stupid business decision. When she realized that her lesson was not about what she earned but about how she had not yet given herself permission to use her creative side, she was free to take some design classes and to make a tentative business plan. This will probably be her big area of growth for a long time, and she can expect periodically to deal with her habit of pulling back into the corporate shell of safety. Creativity is a missing piece in her life puzzle, and it is as alluring as it is frightening.

It is just this push/pull, this combination of lure and resistance, that tells you that you have found a growing edge. The lure will come from your heart. Like a magnet, it will pull you toward what you have been afraid to let in. In spiritual terms, we can say that the heart's longing will draw you toward one of your soul's deepest desires, perhaps your reason for being on the planet in the first place. It's the one lure that you could easily botch because it carries so much weight. It attracts and repels at the same time. If you didn't want it so much, you wouldn't be open to changing your customary mode of operation. This is the tremendous importance of the missing piece. Like the widow's lost coin in the Gospel story, it is what you will sweep the house clean to find. Or at least it's what you want to believe you will sweep the house clean to find. In reality, most of us begin with a little dusting, and then convince ourselves that the thin sliver of a dime found is the gold for which we've been searching. Only when the dime is too quickly spent, do we resume the search. We do this repeatedly, willing to settle for a series of facsimiles as long as we don't really have to tear the house apart in order to find the real thing. This serves to keep fear and effort at bay in the short run, although it is exhausting in the long run. You have probably known the frustration and sadness of jerky starts and stops. Perhaps this is the time when you're ready to pursue the real thing. If you are, you are also committed to doing what it takes to follow where your heart leads you.

A longing of the heart does not indicate something that is permanently unattainable. However, the human mind tends to go in that direction. I will not admit something is wrong, rather than face the possibility that it will be permanently wrong. When I must finally face my longing, I teeter on the brink of despair. But I can hold that longing in my hand like a crystal and examine it from a different angle. Perhaps it is a sign, not of what is impossible, but of what is potentially possible. That potential can be actualized as the energy that is blocked around the longing begins to flow. The gap between potential and actual is not as great as you may think, and speculation about closing that gap has fueled many philosophical and religious debates since time immemorial.

In Mahayana Buddhism for instance, the image of the *garbha* has a twofold meaning. The word is used to mean the womb or container of Buddha-ness, referring to the capacity we all have for nurturing the process of enlightenment. That says the potential is there in each one of us. But the same word is also used to mean the embryo itself contained within the womb which if left untouched will grow to maturity. In that sense, the potential is much more tangible and at some level is already actual. In the Gospels there is constant tension between the reign of God as completely real on some plane we cannot fully comprehend and yet at the same time needing to be made actual through human effort. Every spiritual culture struggles with this, that life already contains everything required and at the same time is perceived by humans as having gaping holes.

To fill the hole which is the perceived lack of love in your own life, you must dip into the reservoir that is already there. One step involves acknowledging the functioning relationships you have just listed as being available. A second step involves creating this kind of relationship everywhere you go. And a third step involves hanging out with folks who have already manifested what you seek.

Let's look at step two. If you have been doing any of the meditative physical, emotional, or spiritual heart openers described in the previous chapters, you may already be watching your relationships with others change. Tapping into that wellspring allows you to approach others non-defensively and can engender a similar response in them, or enable you to understand their limitations without seeing them as judgments on yourself. Even if you have not done many of the other exercises, you can jump in here by experimenting with your everyday encounters.

But first I would encourage you to create an attitude that reminds you of the heart's reality. Make it a practice to periodically breathe into relaxation and check to see whether your posture facilitates the openness described on pages 62–63. Then approach people in your life as if they were going to mirror bits of your highest values and contribute exactly what you need right now in order to learn love's lessons, because in one way or another they will! Give the person before you the support that you desire, knowing that it will come back to you, either from this particular person or from another. You are giving from a fullness that you are in the process of experiencing, however dimly, rather than from a need to get something from the other person. And in the giving, you will generate more activity in the heart chakra. This will feed you from a source far deeper than the person you are addressing.

Knowing that, you will find that your relationships nourish you in new ways. Once you are aware of your own heart, you will be more sensitive to the messages of other hearts. This will enable you to receive what you need from each encounter and leave the rest without recrimination. For instance, when you greet your co-worker with a joyful heart that acknowledges your own strengths and vulnerabilities, you are less likely to take offense at her morning brusqueness. You will understand that there are a multitude of reasons why she may be grumpy, few of which have to do with you. And you'll realize that you don't need her cheer to feed your own joy. So you can give out of fullness and allow your heart's energy to flow. That feels right in itself and may in fact influence the overlapping energy field that is your co-worker. She may never know what happened to alter her mood for the better. If this can happen with a co-worker or a clerk in a store, imagine what can happen with your spouse, child, parent, or best friend! As you remove the chip from your shoulder, the people around you can get closer. And you'll probably find many more people surrounding you as your frequency changes to welcome them.

If your life has room for more nurturing relationships, learn to see every encounter, even the most casual, as a relationship in miniature. Relationships are about giving, and they are also about taking. Even your most important relationships will lack vibrancy until you can take the unique gifts that each offers and appreciate them. You can practice give-and-take wherever you go. Each meeting—a chance encounter, a routine visit to the dentist, a casual dinner date—offers an opportunity to be present with another person, giving what you have and taking a piece of what you need. It may be a smile, a compliment, or a question that invites you to reveal some aspect of yourself that you'd forgotten. Your connection with your own center means you don't expect to get all your needs met in that one occasion, and you can accept that there may be much in that one setting that you don't require. For instance, a woman may find herself in a gentle flirting mode with the piano player at a friend's party. Later on in the evening, she finds out he's gay and is tempted to disregard the whole episode. Why? There was something positive in the interaction and still is if she chooses to accept it. She can choose to both affirm and be affirmed in this, as in any encounter and allow herself and her new friend to feel energized and ready to recreate this kind of vibration in another setting.

A support group offers a more structured way to become aware of interpersonal energy and to work on opening your own blocks. It can be a laboratory for bringing more people into your field and interacting with them in such a way that you are all enriched rather than depleted. A good facilitator can help you notice your blind spots and enable the group to function smoothly. Some of us just don't realize that we're constantly giving advice to others. Instead of saying, "I found this helpful," we say, "You should try..." But even "I found this helpful" gets annoying when repeatedly used. People yearn to be heard compassionately. When we can't do that for very long without trying to fix things, it's time to check in with the heart. The habit of rushing in with words to make things better indicates an unwillingness to feel another's pain and confusion. That happens to me when I don't want to face those same feelings in myself. I'm afraid and, because love and fear cannot cohabit, I need to face my fear in order to be more compassionate. But perhaps you have other tendencies. Maybe you are so unassertive that you fade into the background and no one can tell that you are ready, willing, and able to relate. You may be easily argumentative or so ready to placate and please other people that it is hard to read the true you.

All these styles keep you from others, whether you know it or not. Behavioral changes can bring you closer. Recovery language rightly says, "Fake it until you make it." Acting differently shows you that people will respond to you differently, providing the impetus for you to continue your healing process. But behavioral changes that are only skin deep will not bring lasting transformation. For this, you will want to continue working emotionally, physically, and spiritually on the many levels of yourself revealed by your heart.

But what if you have many supportive personal connections and still desire the one or two that are elusive? You may ache for a mate, or a child to raise, or a close-knit group of friends, or even meaningful work. Those are legitimate yearnings. There is a third way of being with others that assists you in manifesting your heart's desire, and that is simply to hang out with those who have what you want. Some will tell you to avoid this, saying that if you are around too many couples or young families, for instance, you will only increase your misery. If you don't want to know that such happiness really exists because it makes you miserable, then you aren't ready, anyway. Go back a few steps and work on yourself some more. Remember, in spiritual terms, like calls to like. You don't want to covet what anyone else has. Coveting is a no-no in the ten commandments and in the ethics of all traditions because it immediately constricts your heart chakra and takes you off your life track. When you covet anything, you give in to the temptation to believe that someone else's spouse, child, set of friends, lifestyle—whatever—is meant to be yours. But deep down inside you know that you can't live at the center of someone else's circle and be yourself. What you want is your own version of the circle.

After getting past the jealousy, it is easier to see that, if you like the wave that others are riding, it can only help you to hang out at their beach. There's an energy around people who are already creating what you'd like to create. For instance, I share the joys I find in my children and in my work, whether or not those around me are in the same frame of mind. I don't want to pretend that my joys aren't my joys. But I don't brag, and I don't assume that others can't choose the same happiness. Parenthood, for example, is not limited to married people, or to those who can conceive or carry a biological child. I don't know what choices someone may have to make or what barriers they might have to break in order to find their happiness. I just assume it is possible.

Choose to be around the most positive renditions of that which you seek, with people who will welcome you and not consider you either an intrusion or a threat. You want to be around functional families, happy couples, and creative workplaces. If you do otherwise, you will simply absorb other people's tension, and you will probably reinforce any fears and negative feelings you have already. I have several happily married friends whose husbands are dear to me. I feel free to spend time at their house or go out to dinner with the two of them, as free as when I have a partner with me. I enjoy pointing out to each of them what a treasure each has in the other, and I let them know how I benefit by their stability. I can be around their banter without reading any meanings into it, and I am very unobtrusive when a real disagreement occurs. It helps me to tune into couple energy. Then when my girlfriends or clients downplay the possibility of a happy marriage, I remind them of the great couples that I, and probably they, know. If it is possible for some people, I say, it is possible for others. And I remind them that statistics don't count in interpersonal matters. You don't need two hundred perfect prospects from which to choose. You need only one.

Of course, you don't want to spend all your time around others who are already manifesting the energy you seek. You can get so comfortable you may be seduced and give up the time you need to become your best self and to explore the possibilities for manifesting your own creation. If you're with your nieces and nephews so often that you forget to follow up on the appointment with your doctor or call adoption agencies, you are not allowing your process to work for you. You have to be a little uncomfortable with things the way they are in order to be motivated to do the footwork it takes to uncover your options.

A variation on the theme discussed above is to connect, however briefly, with people who are similar to those you could envision attracting. When I am open to a new relationship, there are times when I can't drive past a male toll booth attendant or ask for help from a supermarket clerk without them taking notice. I don't want anything personal from these men. Perhaps because I don't, I feel freer to radiate acceptance. I am quick to express my appreciation for any help they give me. The man who opens the door for me at the mall will, for instance, get a big smile and thank you. The exchange of energy is palpable, and I'm likely to receive a smile or two in return. That's the way energy works. So if you want to meet a good man, never engage in male-bashing. Don't fixate on who hasn't been there for you. Instead, affirm what is good about maleness wherever you find it. This can only serve to harmonize your masculine and feminine energies, thereby preparing you for your own perfect expression of a male partner. The same will hold true for a man, or a woman for that matter, who wants to meet a good woman. Or for the parent wannabe who catches the twinkle in the eye of a little backpack rider at the museum.

Of course, use your street smarts to avoid drawing the attention of a predator or appearing to be one yourself. You are opening your heart for just a second and integrating the results. This is not about playing games, nor about giving or getting unwelcome attention. It is about expanding your field to affirm and include the pieces that are missing from your experience. It is about raising the frequency with which you meet another's vibration. It is about positive calling to positive.

Remember to continue the psychological and spiritual work that makes you ready for what comes. You'll want to spend time with special friends, with advisers and guides, and with yourself. This last piece is crucial, for there must be enough time and space for you to let your imagination soar. You can't possibly create what you can't even imagine. Sometimes your dreams will do the imagining for you, so be sure to pay attention to them. Just before I conceived my first child, my dreams began to be filled with beautiful babies. One in particular I still remember as being surrounded by a golden light. I knew this was my child-to-be, although I had not rationally made the choice to have one.

At another time in my life I'd been wondering whether I'd even know how to form a healthy emotional tie. I'd been married and had lots of relationships, but they'd all come from logic or lust rather than from love, from upper chakra shoulds or lower chakra desires instead of from the heart. Then my dreams took over. They became filled with warm, healthy, romantic encounters in which I gave and received support, felt safe yet intrigued, and had lots of fun. Even then I knew what was happening and marveled in my journal that I was being prepared to recognize what I'd not had a chance to experience. Then I had a session with an intuitive counselor who understood my dilemma and suggested that we go into a meditative state so that I could take in the male approval and love he would radiate. I didn't put much stock in the exercise but figured it couldn't hurt. Within three months, I'd met the person with whom I'd be intensely involved for the next couple of years. He was the one from whom I learned how loved and loving I could be, and this was the relationship that prepared me for true partnership. Ironically, I realized after our engagement that he could not sustain a commitment and also realized that I had indeed been gifted with my counselor's energy. He and my ex-fiancé shared significant characteristics and vital statistics, not all of them positive.

That experience provided confirmation that this energy work is real and powerful. See yourself in a magical laboratory with glass tubes bubbling all around you. The combinations are endless and you are the chemist, willing to experiment and learn. Once you stop playing and fix on one combination, you can manipulate the substances so that everything happens just the way you expect. But when you surrender to the alchemist who is working through you, this laboratory, your life, becomes a place of miracles where anything is possible.

CHOOSING FROM CLARITY

Dissension within families, the burgeoning number of divorces, the rate at which business partnerships fail—all speak to the fragility of human relationships. Perhaps our biggest mistake is in denying that fragility. When awareness moves out of the heart and that chakra ceases to spin merrily, even a mild difference of opinion can turn into a battle of wills. And with the variety of motives, desires, opinions, and feelings that drive us on an ordinary day, it's a wonder that any of us get along at all. So it's wise to consider our relationships as an intrinsic part of spiritual practice.

Spiritual practice requires intention combined with self-discipline and work. When we neglect this process, the possibility that growth will come out of normal disagreement between people is severely diminished. The exercises in this book have been designed to help you bring awareness to the heart chakra, a key mover of relationship energy. Doing them regularly increases the likelihood that you'll stay open in the heart chakra even when you find yourself engaged in a dispute.

Sometimes it seems as if the easiest way to take your awareness *out* of the heart chakra is by forming an alliance with another human being. "But how can that be?" you counter, "Don't we form attachments because of a longing in the heart?" It's true—that may be the initial impetus. Under the best of circumstances, it is love that calls us to begin friendships, to enter romantic partnerships, to become parents, and to align with supportive colleagues in order to accomplish meaningful work. You'll recognize it as love because it is such an immediate and intense creative force. You have uncovered a piece of your soul's desire. But what begins as an awakening of the soul becomes an emotional investment. You're hooked, and at first the immersion is so complete that it is almost a meditation in itself. You've fallen in love and into the present moment. And as long as you're intent on staying awake, all of this can be part of the spiritual practice. However, once you are more committed to preserving what was so fulfilling rather than to meeting it in the here and now, you've fallen out of the moment and into illusion. You've actually fallen out of love although you may not realize it for a long time. The heartbeat is the physical reminder of an energy that must continually flow. If you're attached to the person you knew yesterday or projecting the person you will know tomorrow, you are not loving the one in front of you today, even if all three carry the same name and Social Security number.

It's an eye-opener to sit with a couple who have been happily married for ten years. Now they are having trouble and don't understand why things have become so difficult. The husband wants to leave his lucrative salaried job in order to start a new business. This means the wife will have to go back to work sooner than she liked. She worries about the effect of her doing so on their child and also mourns the loss of her freedom. This is a time of push and pull that threatens to turn into a tug-of-war. All he's asking of her is to see him for who he is today instead of who he was a year ago. But he needs to realize that this is a huge request in a marriage where the roles have suited both of them for so long. This could be a major turning point in the evolution of their relationship, allowing them to move from being husband and wife to being spiritual partners. Whether that happens does not depend on which solution they choose or their ability to modify their roles. A marriage counselor can help them compromise and redefine their roles without facilitating a major shift in either person's consciousness. This shift will come about only if they agree to make it a habit to look past their habits and roles. They have to make a commitment to breathe together into each new moment as it arises. This frees the heart center to process energy and generate true love that isn't based on fear or control.

A situation like that faced by this couple is an opportunity to practice non-attachment. Why is it so difficult? Practicing non-attachment means accepting that life is about change when we'd much rather cling to the myth of constancy. Most of us will fight to maintain the status quo before trying something new. Like you, I don't change easily. When I do, it can feel as if the rug has been pulled out from under me. My ego, fearing its final demise, holds on for dear life and tries to stay attached to what it thinks is safe. To be honest, I can't blame it. It's only doing what an ego is supposed to do, and so far it's done a pretty good job of keeping me alive and functional. But without spiritual practice, it's too afraid to do its work creatively. My ego cares about survival, and as far as it's concerned, survival is about casting the play and doing whatever it takes to ensure a long run. It will encourage, cajole, beg, or force all the actors to perform their parts. It doesn't want to know about improvisation. The scene as scripted is all important. But a fixed script imprisons souls.

A lingerie boutique on a trendy street in Philadelphia has a window sign that reads something like: "Love hurts. Your intimate apparel shouldn't. Let us fit you." Every time I see it, I wonder how many of the people walking by have their attention captured because they agree with that first sentence. Many of us have experienced the pain associated with love, especially in the process of coupling and uncoupling. But is it the love that hurts, or is it something else? If love is the product of the appropriate opening of the heart chakra, then love itself cannot hurt. But it's common to confuse love with other drives and emotions. When I experience excessive activity or blockage in one of the other energy centers while I'm relating to another person for whom there is some attraction, the simplest solution is to label what I'm feeling as love. For example, if I haven't kept in close contact with how heart energy feels when it's flowing, I may imagine that my thoughts of duty and obligation are being generated in the heart, even though they are coming from the unbalanced upper chakras. Or I may imagine that the lust or dependency I feel is coming from the heart, even though they are coming from unbalanced lower chakras. But when I stay in touch with the heart through breath work, yoga, and meditation it's harder to be misled and I'm saved a lot of unnecessary tears. In fact, I've found that there's an inverse proportion between the depth of love and the number of tears shed. On a normal day, love does not make you cry.

You ask me, "What about the genuine love I feel for someone who makes bad choices?" First I'd ask who the person is. If it's your significant other who consistently makes choices that are bad for his own well-being and yours as well, the situation needs to be evaluated from that perspective. Love doesn't mean routinely risking your physical, emotional, or financial health. If you don't make appropriate choices for yourself, the love itself will devolve. The lack of give-and-take between you and your significant other will sap your energy over time. You will constantly be giving from your stock of energy, compulsively thinking about, praying for, or beseeching your lover, or intervening in his life. You can sense the imbalance. If you check in by placing your hand on your heart during one of these episodes, you'll find very little warmth and light emanating from there. You might feel a knot in your stomach or a throbbing in your head. Any of these symptoms could give you the information you need to make choices. Sometimes the love persists but the partnership needs to change or dissolve. One reason we don't check in regularly is that there's a lot we really don't want to know.

Of course, there are other persons for whom it is appropriate to do more; for instance, a teen-aged child whom you suspect to be engaged in petty crime or flirting with drugs. However, it is still helpful to be able to differentiate between your heart-felt sadness over the behavior of your child and the impulses that arise within you about changing that behavior. The latter must be weighed against the former if you are to decide from compassion rather than from a need to fix or control. You could be angry because your child lied to you, or embarrassed because you wanted to save face. Neither of these reactions comes from the heart chakra. No intervention on your part that stems from sources such as these is likely to be successful in the long run. The bond between you and your child presupposes two separate but overlapping fields with a unique evolution for each. No two people walk the exact same path, which is easy to say but hard to live. Sometimes a person, even a parent, must simply watch and pray as a child hits bottom, a bottom that may be more cavernous than the one standing guard hopes. You may "save" your child over and over again, but if he doesn't learn the crucial lessons that are meant to be his, the purpose of his experiences will not have been served. Then, as the same behavior continues in one form or another, your baffled question will probably be, "Haven't you learned anything from this?" You'll be overwhelmed by the realization that love hurts. However, this won't be completely accurate.

What hurts is not the love but the letting go that love sometimes requires. We fear letting go because we fear loss; but, in fact, loss is always a component when we love on the physical plane. Even when we are not changing, growing, and walking away from each other, death awaits its day. Knowing this, we connect letting go with the end of love rather than with the process of love and do whatever we can to avoid it. It's hard to recognize separation as a necessary step in the dance of intimacy, but that's what it is. How can you appreciate coming back together with someone unless you have felt free to whirl away? How can the other? Ancient wisdom has always advised to hold with relaxed hands that which you love and to let it fly if it will. Only when it comes back to you do you know something more definite about the relationship. Do this consistently and you begin to make of love a spiritual discipline, because a spiritual discipline by definition includes the practice of non-attachment. Do you imagine that being non-attached means being uncaring or noncommittal? Non-attachment is rich with commitment—your own. It does not presume to know ahead of time what the other's commitment might be or how it will play out. And it is commitment to the process of relating rather than to some end point. It's a bit like driving on the expressway. I know where I'm heading, and having a destination is a good thing. But I can never predict with complete certainty that I will arrive at my destination at the appointed time using only the planned route. Yet I often drive as if I could. Then, when changes are called for, I get far angrier than when I've allowed myself some psychological leeway (and maybe an extra half hour) to make those changes. Holding on to my ideas about the particulars of the destination can make getting there very unpleasant for me and those with whom I travel. How many of us see relationship as destination rather than journey? How many marriages can claim longevity as their only reward? That happens when spouses are more committed to the accumulation of anniversaries than to the exploration and discovery of each other's unique set of needs. They'll make it to their fortieth anniversary (or so at least one of them assumes) even if it kills them! I know the feeling. But even when I think that I am focusing on the journey instead of the destination, I can still trip myself up when I decide ahead of time how everyone else on the road must behave. For instance, it does me no good to synchronize my speed with the moving traffic a half mile in front of me. If the car in front of me decides to brake suddenly, I'd better notice. It doesn't matter whether that driver has a good reason or not to do this. While I want to retain a peripheral awareness of the entire highway, my immediate attention needs to be on the bumper directly in front of me or I'm setting myself up for a crash.

Many of us go through life completely unaware of the collisions waiting to happen. We're either focused inwardly on our own needs and drives or outwardly on some solution we've found to fulfill them. When that solution involves another person or set of people, it's as if they have no autonomy. We see only what we want to see. When one of the others no longer likes what's happening and tries to voice that but is not heard, the brakes may be put on abruptly. What happens next may seem like a complete surprise but need not have been. Think of a young adult who carries the weight of what his parents want him to be. They want only the best for him, and he knows that. What he doesn't know, even in college, is where they end and he begins. If, as a family they have developed no language with which to discuss his plans, he may see escape as his only option. His parents will not be aware that anything is wrong until they get a call from the dean to inform them that he has dropped out of school, with his current whereabouts unknown. These parents will commiserate with other parents about how painful it is to love an ungrateful child. However, the love wasn't what caused the pain. Their unwillingness to allow him to be more than a bit player in their script and their failure to notice when he was unhappy playing the role made it necessary for him to quit school in order to write his script. They believed their commitment was to him, but it was really to some entity that may be called parenthood. That's not the kind of heartfelt commitment that calls forth the best in another person.

It is not love that brings pain but rather the melodrama that is created around love. And the melodrama is not a necessary component, for it's not really about love at all. It's not about the energy of the heart. It is about blocked or excessive energy in one of the other chakras. You create a melodrama when you fixate rather than dialogue. Fixation takes you out of the heart and traps you elsewhere in your energy field. If you won't let go of an idea of how someone or some relationship must look, regardless of what's really happening, you're staying in the upper realms. If you're hanging on to someone no matter what, because it keeps you from examining your fear of being alone, you're staying in the lower realms. The bottleneck is closed, and others around you will sense the imbalance even if they can't name it and will likely respond from their own imbalances. You will know that something's wrong, even if you can't admit it. A story will begin to develop around your particular set of circumstances, and you'll recognize the characters you meet and become: the rejected lover, the ungrateful child, the unappreciated colleague, the abandoned friend, the savior, etc., etc. Soon that story will seem more real than anything else and you will vibrate to its frequency, developing the plot as you go. It takes on a life of its own as you allow it to become a melodrama.

We're all vulnerable to this in one area of life or another. My growing edge has shown up in the area of romance. I was always able to be conscious in my work life. As my awareness deepened over the years, I also found myself developing into an invested, but non-attached mom and friend. But for a long time romance was the hook. In my early years I chose so inappropriately for myself that I could have written the dramatic plots on day one if I'd been willing to see what was really going on. I progressed to choosing more appropriately but failing to keep abreast of current developments. I still wound up in the same predicament, but my lead time was growing. Whereas before I could sustain a long relationship based on five minutes of positive interaction during a dinner date, now I would insist on five months or even a year's worth of positive interaction. With that under my belt, I could still manage to avoid noticing when the person stopped meeting me in the moment and retreated into well-worn coping mechanisms that had nothing to do with me. That's what happened with the man whom I was engaged to, but didn't marry. We began with a real emotional connection that for the first time opened my heart chakra in a romantic way. But he had no ability to speak his truth and I had no desire to notice and ruin the fairy tale. Together we created a structure called "us" that did not involve discussing the differences between "you" and "me." As I struggled to uphold that structure built on sand, my fairy tale rapidly deteriorated into a melodrama of the first order.

Could I have recognized our differences in values and communication styles before the bitter end that so "surprised" me? Of course, in theory. But in practice I needed to do it one more time—this time with heart—so I could understand that entering the drama meant leaving the heart space. What begins as love may not continue as that, for how can you love the person you are willing to ignore?

After the worst of my sadness passed, I counseled a young woman who'd just been left by her boyfriend of several years. She had the kind of limp hair and tearstained face I'd seen in my own mirror just months before. Wringing her hands, she told of all the ways in which he'd pulled away from her in the past months and how she'd pretended not to see or told herself it would pass. In fact, she was still using up precious energy in pretending. She couldn't quite admit the importance of what she was saying. "But he was perfect for me," she wailed. Was he? I repeated to her several of the aspects of their life together that she'd just told me, revealing major differences and incompatibilities over a long period of time. A look of comprehension washed over her. Of course, she still had months of depression and self-doubt ahead of her, but at that moment her healing began. She started to see the drama for what it was. He was not her last, best hope for marriage and children, even though he may have been her most compatible romantic partner thus far. Her ideal partnership would be one which did not require delusion in order to sustain itself. But first she would have to commit to staying with her own process. She would have to love herself as well as she desired to be loved by another.

We invent princes and princesses as rescuers because we don't love ourselves enough. We accept shoddy behavior in the name of commitment and try to become rescuers because we don't love ourselves enough. One of my clients is a recovering alcoholic who is firmly committed to her recovery program. After years of turmoil she is developing a supportive network of sponsors and friends. She has given up her lucrative job of bartending and waitressing because they were dangerous for her sobriety and got some special training to become an administrator. She is working hard to develop clear communication with her three young sons, who have been with her through the ups and downs and suffer from their own sets of problems. But she does not really believe that she's entitled to a peaceful life, so there has to be a fly in the ointment. In this case, it's her second husband, a childish man who keeps reverting to his addiction. Just when finances, family communication, and work satisfaction all seem to be coming together, she discovers some way in which he has sabotaged their life. Sometimes he uses drugs or alcohol, sometimes he wrecks their budget by overspending, sometimes he is verbally abusive to her or the boys. She threatens to put him out, at least until he gets sober; but, since she never follows through on her threats, he doesn't take them seriously and continues his behavior. "I've already let one marriage go down the tubes. Shouldn't

I work on this one?" she asks me. Because she equates working on a relationship with taking abuse, she would have to deal with her own guilt if she were to set clear boundaries. She hasn't yet accepted that she deserves a partner and not a project because she hasn't yet allowed herself to experience the fullness of divine love working within her.

Telling someone to love herself is both wisdom and a cliché. Whenever I've heard that advice, my train of thought has gone something like this: "Well, I like myself well enough most of the time and value myself and think I'm worth inviting good things into my life. But is that love? I know that love isn't only a feeling, but it has to include feeling. What does loving myself feel like? Love has a quality of gift to it. I certainly treat myself from time to time, but that doesn't have the same delightful quality as someone surprising me with a present. No matter how I define it, love has something of otherness about it. Where's the power in little old me loving little old me?"

But it isn't just little old me loving little old me! It is little old me (my ego) receiving love from the me (my soul) connected to a far deeper source. In that sense, it is not quite true that I am loving myself. I prefer to say that I am allowing my soul to love me. The soul makes itself known through the heart chakra, and when that opens in you, you are the first recipient of its generous activity. It feels wonderful, as if a fist inside your chest had unclenched to radiate warm sunlight in the winter. So it is no platitude to say that you must love your neighbor as yourself. There is some variation of that bit of wisdom in most of the cultures of the world, and it's there for a reason. It's there because the experience of being loved—or of loving yourself, if you will—does not depend on circumstance, but is universal and available to all. You are not being advised to love from a state of emptiness but rather from fullness. That fullness is retrievable through the energy center known everywhere by different names, some of them being the fourth chakra, the tiferet, the sacred heart of Jesus, and the compassionate heart of the bodhisattva. If you are having a hard time drawing on this energy within your personal experience, an array of saints, both alive and deceased, who embody its qualities are available to you. They eagerly await your association and identification with them, and have entered our pantheon for this very reason. By opening the reality of love to you, they continue their existence of loving service.

Once you have learned to love yourself from this deeper perspective, you will never again so easily mistake abuse for love. You will neither want to abuse nor be abused and you will step away from any such situation. In so doing, you will not be saying that you are unwilling to work on a particular relationship. You will merely be saying that you are not willing to demean what spirit loves. When I struggled with old feelings around my former fiancé and considered revisiting what I knew to be a relationship grown toxic, my spiritual advisor asked, "Why wish pain on yourself?" The fog lifted, and I realized that any sorrow that would come out of further interaction would be of my own choosing.

How little could I value myself to be the one to inflict my own pain? That's the gift, and the responsibility of consciousness. Now I use that question whenever I am tempted to forego my best long-term development for a taste of short-term gratification. Why would I wish pain on myself? Why would you?

If the person or group from whom you have stepped away rethinks their position and approaches you with a new agenda, you always have the right to step in again. You do not leave with anger or recrimination. You leave as a symbol of the value you attach to your own well-being. You may want to make some statement to that effect so that others have a chance to mull it over. But words don't work unless you follow through with action. The action can be as small or large as the transgression. Action toward a group at work telling disturbing jokes might mean a walk to the copy machine to get away from them. Toward an abrasive family it might mean having Thanksgiving dinner with friends this year. Toward an abusive spouse it might mean a move toward separation and possible divorce. There are no rules carved in stone. It's always your choice. Is sacrifice sometimes called for? Of course. The greatest people have always made the biggest sacrifices. But they did not make them unconsciously or without guidance. The people I know who remain in unrewarding or downright abusive situations are staying out of weakness rather than out of nobility. If you are going to put your life on the line, do it for some great purpose and with full awareness. Don't allow yourself to be pecked to death by ducks in the name of self-sacrifice. You will still die, and the ducks will have learned nothing.

You can only love yourself, that is, allow your soul to love you, in the present moment. Choosing love means continuing to be in the present, because it is only in the present that you can be completely yourself. When you run from yourself, you run to the past or future, and therein lies the drama. In order to see yourself as you were, or as you'd like to be, you must skew the way you look at your situation and the people around you. Of course, it's a gift to be a visionary and to see life for what it could be. But that never means closing your eyes to what it is right now. Too often we see what we want to see and say that's because we're looking for the best in everyone when it's really because we're avoiding the truth. My teenager is not promiscuous, my spouse doesn't drink too much, my employer will give me that promotion right after this next project is completed. I remember one attractive woman sitting in my office years ago, complaining that she usually attracted a ne'er-do-well kind of man. "I meet someone, and I can just tell how much he'd have to offer if he'd just shape up," she said, "so I give him a chance. Aren't we supposed to see the good in people?" "You can help as many people as you'd like," I counseled, "but you don't have to date them, and you certainly shouldn't marry them. Personal relationship is not social work." She was stunned. Somehow, she'd never thought of that. Within a couple of years she was happily married to an equal partner instead of one of her projects.

Love yourself enough to drop out of the struggles you create around relationship. At its source, love is the pure joy that sustains through the ups and downs we all experience. Things happen, and life will contain enough sorrow just by virtue of your living it on the physical plane. People will disappoint you because they are human. People will move away. People will die. This is all hard enough when we're breathing into the present moment of the heart space. When we stop breathing, so to speak, it all becomes that much harder and the struggle begins. Life for many of us resembles gasping for air. We say we'd like to clear our lungs, but, in fact, we'd hardly be able to recognize ourselves without the struggle. It feels familiar, and it keeps us from having to make difficult choices. Love yourself, and then love the person(s) in front of you. In so doing, you will love appropriately, rather than dramatically. That means you will not stand for bad behavior today just because you didn't notice it yesterday and it might go away tomorrow. When you sidestep the drama and struggle that block the flow of heart chakra energy, you are not avoiding intimacy. You are freeing up your relationships to be the best that they can be. You are actually giving love a chance.

THE NEW CREATION

Just as your life is your soul's own creation, so the larger world is our joint creation. A world in which many starve while a few take far more than their share is our creation. So is a world in which children become so angry after only eight years on the planet that they shoot and kill other children. The reasons for such horrors are many and complex, and the solutions are too. On the most basic level, however, it is possible to state with absolute certainty that we have such a world because as a species we are not acting from an open heart chakra.

The Adam, the Christ, the Buddha as Bodhisattva—they represent every individual who separately carries the divine spark, as well as that collective entity we form together as human consciousness. It is our shared consciousness that determines how much of the source energy is being manifested at any moment in the world as we know it.

Imagine humanity with all its potential in the shape of your own body, then overlay a diagram of the various pathways energy may travel around your body. At its center will always be the integrator, the harmonizer, the transmuter. On the physical plane, this looks like the organ you call your heart. On the emotional level, it feels like an opening or closing response to various beings and situations. On the collective level, it is the pulsing of the ultimate creative vibration that is the primal expression of love.

You did not get here by accident; you got here by love, and that is true whether or not your biological parents loved each other or you. We've seen that the nature of Ultimate Reality is love. Any impulse of that nature to move from unity to diversity stems from a desire to experience intimate relationship with its own creation—and that means you and me! We've seen that devotion to the Sacred carries the power to soften the heart because it positions us within an intimate relationship that allows us to admit need and acknowledge guidance. But, truth be told, devotion doesn't start on this end. Spiritual traditions have always taught that we love because we are first loved. In reality, the Sacred is devoted to you from the very first moment that your individuality is imagined.

The more frequently we as individuals acknowledge this and tune into the vibration of love, the stronger it will grow in our collective awareness. It's like my pulse that I have to make an effort to notice. When my aerobics instructor calls for a pulse at the beginning, middle, and end of class, I have to stop for a moment and remember how to take it. Then— there it is again, rhythmic and strong.

We can also learn to take the pulse of the collective body. We can learn to become aware of those moments when we are clearly functioning well as part of a larger organism. We need that experience, and when we find it, our joy knows no bounds. This is one reason for the proliferation of drumming circles in the past decade. Through this shared activity that requires little training, it is possible to experience what words cannot express. Before I signed up for a drumming workshop with Babatunde Olatunji, the Nigerian-born sage and master, I wondered whether I would stay attentive through the week I signed up for. While I registered eagerly, I silently gave myself permission to pursue any other interest that might call to me. To my surprise, however, I never wanted to leave. The drums called to me over and over again. Whether I was actively playing my drum, sitting with my eyes closed absorbing the vibration, or participating in the African dance sequences, I was captivated. The shared rhythm echoed my own personal rhythm, and I felt my being expand to encompass it. Even at break time or at the end of the day, it was difficult to tear myself away. To do so was to tear myself away from the heartbeat of the universe, to separate myself voluntarily from vitality itself.

In our modern world, there is a hum of energy just beneath the surface of life. Stop, breathe, and listen. Do you hear the drone of the countless refrigerators, televisions, computers, and phones? You're used to tuning them out. Silence is not really silence anymore. But keep breathing even past that and you will sometimes find something deeper. It's the throb of creation that is our connection to divinity. Instruments like the drum and the didgeridoo participate in that primal heartbeat so wondrously that they bring us energy from the source. They are instruments of healing. Are we?

When my daughter played the flute in her high school and college marching bands, I got a little closer to the world of cooperative sound. Amy had to practice by herself and with others for many hours a week in order to create music that would stir the crowds at the football game on Saturday night. In addition, she had to pay a lot of attention to her flute. As her skill improved, she required a better flute. Prior to her acquiring that second, more finely crafted flute, I didn't understand how much the quality of an instrument affected the sound. Of course, she also needed to keep it clean and polished. Her flute was her conduit, the channel for her breath, and it needed to be kept open, free of gunk.

St. Francis asked God in a prayer to make him an instrument of divine peace. Indeed, we are also instruments. Breath passes in, out, and through us. We are channels of spirit by virtue of our energetic makeup. Yet many of us resist being called channels because it sounds scary, esoteric, or blasphemous. But our chakras vibrate as feeling, color, and sound; and we as conscious beings can choose the quality of the feelings, the brightness of the colors, the clarity of the sounds. You can choose to be an open, clean conduit. This happens when the issues of each chakra are processed in a spiritual way, whether the techniques used are mental, physical, emotional, or aesthetic. When in doubt, begin with the heart and use some of the practices in this book. Remember that the health of the heart is an indicator of the well-being of the whole system and that, when the heart chakra is functional, the whole system has an enhanced opportunity to flow smoothly.

As your heart chakra opens, you will receive love from your soul. As you bask in that love, you will not be content to remain a mere recipient of such largesse. You will be as concerned for the well-being of those around you as for your own well-being. Ultimately, you will become just as concerned for the well-being of those far away from you, geographically or emotionally, and for the well-being of creation as a whole. Then you may recognize that you are not only evolving, but contributing to the evolution of the human species and the expansion of consciousness on the planet. You will see yourself as the "Everyone," and this will engender an attitude of surrender rather than arrogance, for it will be about soul rather than ego. In that brief instant in which you become identified with the Adam, the Christ, the Bodhisattva, you become the overlay on the body of the world. Your own healing manifests and contributes to the healing of all that lives, including the earth itself.

We have created a world broken by our own inability to surrender in this way. In fixating on the individual self, we damage our individual heart that wants to reflect the larger soul and, in so doing, become an arrhythmia in the cosmic heartbeat. Acknowledging this, the Jewish people encourage a state of being called *tikkun*, the repairing of the broken creation through human activity. A true *mitzvah*, sometimes translated as a good deed, is an action that contributes to tikkun. For instance, when you give food or money to another person who is in need, you align your deed with life's best impulses. The harmony thus created is not limited to the helper and person who is being helped—it helps attune the physical cosmos to the highest vibration. On some mystical level where the seen and the unseen are one reality, it can be said that the unraveled fibers of the tapestry of life get rewoven and the regularity of the cosmic heartbeat is restored. So what the Christians have taught—that the sacrificial act of one person can benefit many—is true. It is also true, as the Mahayana Buddhists have noted, that the people who take full responsibility for their own enlightenment ultimately realize the futility of trying to retreat into nirvana alone. It is not nirvana unless and until all of us are transformed.

We are moving together into a transformation of consciousness itself. Teilhard de Chardin, the mid-twentieth century mystic/paleontologist/theologian, described this as a journey of the species toward the evolutionary Omega point. At that point we will be one with each other in awareness and joined with divine intention. He used the human heart to symbolize this new creation, since it is characterized by conscious love rather than by pure intellect. Of course, this seems like just another working hypothesis. Most of us cannot even imagine how any one group of humans, never mind the whole species, could manage to work in unison with each other or share the job of leading the group for more than a few minutes. But we need not let the vastness of the goal keep us from the process. The issue for each of us here and now is direct and particular: "What am I doing to jumpstart or flow with this evolutionary process?" There are lots of tasks to be done, lots of ideas to mull over, and lots of spiritual practices to try. It's easy to be confused about how to contribute, but an old saying is worth mentioning here: "It's not enough to look around the world and pick something that needs to be done. Rather, pray to discern what piece of the work is being given to you by God as your own."

It is arrogant to try to do it all. This presumes that no one else has the ability or desire to pick up the slack. It is futile to run from one task to the next as requests or demands come your way. This presumes that you are at the beck and call of outside forces. It is wasteful of your gifts to stay with a task for which you feel no talent or interest. This presumes that what inspires and enthuses you can be of no use to the world and that only drudgery is valid. Joseph Campbell's words encourage us to follow our bliss. This advice assumes that what and how you choose to contribute is important, for as you evolve, so does the species. If you choose love and joy, you are embodying these qualities in yourself. This is not a selfish act. You are embodying them in yourself, but not merely for yourself. In actuality, you are imprinting them on the whole of human experience in your own unique way. What you choose, good or bad, we all use; and what you don't choose, good or bad, we all lose. Spiritual evolution means that your decisions affect not only yourself and those around you but also those at a distance and those who have yet to be born.

As we become more conscious, we begin to notice that evolution has a definite feel to it. It's a deep-seated sense of rightness combined with an intellectual assent, with the blend not centered in the gut or in the head, but in the heart. Every one of us gets such a feeling at least once in a while, but few of us can recognize it often enough and with enough certainty to make a habit of following its guidance. Learn to notice what's going on, as we've done in exercises such as taking the heart's temperature, and you can more easily tune into and trust your own feelings.

I teach yoga in a variety of settings. I try to choose quiet places. Some are dedicated to yoga and meditation, while others are multi-purpose. It's always a luxury to be in a yoga studio dedicated to the practice with everything provided that might be needed, but the multi-purpose setting is its own gift. At one such place, an adult education center, I had a revelation as I left the room for a brief moment while my students lay in *sevasana*, the resting pose after the other postures. Behind me were a dozen people lying flat out on the floor, their bodies loose, their minds free to wander. Soft music played in the background. The atmosphere was relaxed, yet charged with the focus and effort of the last hour. Contained within that cocoon, it was easy to forget the world outside. But as soon as I opened the door, the very air seemed different, and this took me by surprise. I've become used to sensing obvious environmental differences. Like me, you may notice that you can tell from the vibes of a room whether it's been the scene of happy or sad encounters. But in this case I was not leaving "good" and entering "bad." I was merely moving from a yoga class into the larger waiting area with a reception desk and telephone. Across the hall, people worked, setting up future classes, and next door the teacher was going on about financial planning. It is a congenial place, and I love walking through the building on the mornings I teach there. But, in an instant, I was able to experience the dramatic contrast between ordinary and extraordinary consciousness. The energy outside the yoga room was jangled, and even the calmest people doing ordinary things there seemed to be affected by it. I was affected by it and quickly finished my errand, returning gratefully to my class. As I closed the door behind me and watched the blissful faces that emerged from resting, I related my experience and reminded them of the tremendous luxury we enjoy and the responsibility we share.

In this time and place, it is so easy to slide into hedonism. And even when we are not over-indulging, it's easy to sink into energy-sapping guilt. But I often tell my students that there's a responsible way to use the resources we've been given in the twenty-first century in middle class North

America. The only justification for being born here and now is to contribute to the evolution of awareness. When we regularly attune our vibration to a higher frequency, we are doing just that. Together we can create the bliss of the yoga room everywhere. We can unseal its doors and windows so that its peacefulness seeps into the nooks and crannies of the outer office and blurs the difference between the two spaces.

It is not just those people who have no commitment to our common evolution who are failing to do their part—it is also those whose commitment is other than heart-centered. Have you run into people who are so sure their cause is right? It is virtually impossible to have a conversation in which they don't try to convert you to their side. I have. I've met pacifists whose inner turmoil became evident the moment I questioned a particular aspect of their strategy to attain lasting world peace. I've gone to dinner with people who defined themselves as vegetarians and refused to eat anything on their plates because some animal product might have tainted their food. They preferred to insult their host rather than loosen up, self-righteously rejecting what was offered in good faith. We're used to thinking of idealistic people as good people, but idealism must walk hand-in-hand with compassion to have integrity.

Recognize that such rigid people exist, but don't judge them too harshly. If you do, you are playing by their rules. And that hurts. Instead of judging, empathize with them silently. Then move your awareness inside yourself to locate your own places of rigidity. You'll recognize them by the emotions and body sensations they engender. As you mull over a particular idea or commitment of yours, notice whether your body clamps down or your feelings shut down. Isolate the place in the body that feels tight and invite it to loosen with some deep, regular breaths. Pay attention to a subtle pain or tension that is barely noticeable. For some people merely beginning to think about a particular issue leads to an intense headache or upset stomach. But they don't pay attention to such clues because noticing them might mean having to make some changes. It seems easier to ignore the symptoms rather than to put two and two together. Don't do that. Notice the signals you're getting physically and emotionally. When you talk about feeding the hungry, are you willing to feel their hunger in your belly and their abandonment in your heart? Or are you most often engulfed by rage at the system that allows hunger to happen, or at your colleagues who never do enough to ease the situation? Righteous anger is one of the emotions you may experience, but it cannot be the only one, or the primarily motivating one. What is causing you or those around you discomfort? Why are you afraid to listen to another opinion or imagine a different scenario? Remember, you don't have to change anything—outlook or behavior—but if you're unwilling to examine the possibility of change, it's unlikely that your stance is held from a position of love. Non-attachment and true love always walk hand-in-hand.

The vibration of the heart chakra is the color green, and those who see such things know that the color green is not a theory but a reality. They also report that people who habitually live according to their heart's guidance have an aura that is suffused in a rosy glow. We used to laugh at those who see the world through rose-colored glasses. Turns out it's the only way to see the world as it really is. Through these glasses, you will also see where your compassion can best serve. Then you can give without comparing yourself to others. Don't be intimidated by those doing big things—the organizers, the politicians, the writers, and the teachers, the activists and the public figures. Understand that their merit is not in what they do, but in why and how they do it. And so is yours.

You are the first recipient of your soul's love when your heart chakra opens, but you are never its only recipient. Loving yourself, or allowing your soul to love you, is not a selfish experience. It sets the stage for you to water the earth from a fountain that never runs dry. If it's coming from the center, the smallest teardrop is as effective as a waterfall. Handing a sandwich to a hungry person can be the same as starting a food bank. In either case, of course, someone in need will be an immediate beneficiary. But the long-term benefits to your own spiritual well-being and that of humanity's evolution will depend more on motivation than on the numbers of people affected. Spirit is no statistician. Spirit registers the most subtle vibrational shift as if it were cataclysmic.

So acclimate yourself to your center. Let your heart chakra open to process upper and lower energies and transmute them into love. Know what that feels like so you can encourage it to happen more often with the meditations and exercises in this book. Experience self-love and then pass it on. Do some things and refrain from others. Give money to the person in the street who asks for help, even though you may suspect the money may be spent for liquor or drugs. Or simply ask the person what he or she would like to eat, take the order, buy it, and present it. Don't participate in conversations that disparage other people. See if the agenda of some community-minded group speaks to you enough to join it or at least make a contribution. Tread lightly on the earth, and recognize that it, too, is alive. Let that awareness encourage you to make small changes in the way you shop, recycle, or conserve energy. Don't do these things to be politically correct. Act from the heart, and your vibration will quicken and move outward into an ever-expanding circle that encompasses the whole planet. You're giving in some places and receiving in others, creating in your microcosm what seems overwhelming to imagine on the grand scale. Check in periodically with your heart to make sure your activity is being generated from there. Then you'll know that your desire to repair the world comes from your willingness to repair your relationship with soul. If you're feeling tight and tense, it's time to soften before trying to do more. Unless you are in the midst of earthquake or flood, don't ignore your feelings and push on. Life is a process, not an emergency.

Life is what it feels like. If it consistently feels difficult, that's not because life is supposed to be that way. It's because you are regularly choosing duty, laziness, or avoidance over love. Love is not always easy and sometimes requires hard choices and sacrifice. But it is not a constant grit-your-teeth, nose-to-the-grindstone experience. Taking care of a sick spouse or child, for example, has a totally different quality depending whether you're doing it from obligation or from compassion. The former hardens the caregiver, and this edge can be felt by the one receiving help. The latter softens the caregiver and heals the one receiving help. By extension, it also heals the world. The activity is the same; the motivation is different.

If our twenty-first century society feels alienating and stressful, it is. And it can be remedied. The feeling is not a sign of what has to be but a sign of what needs healing. As the activation of the personal heart chakra is balm to the frazzled individual, so the activation of the cosmic heart is balm to the broken world. This is what the mystics of Judaism, Christianity, Buddhism, and other spiritual traditions have always known. This is the old wisdom that the new science is now recognizing when it acknowledges energy as the wave that sustains life. Claim it for your own and your life will change. Love will no longer be just the stuff of songs and movies. It will be the stuff that you are made of.

OTHER BOOKS BY THE CROSSING PRESS

Black Holes and Energy Pirates: How to Recognize and Release Them

By Jesse Reeder

Two phenomena that keep people from reaching their natural creative potential are black holes—unconscious patterns, expectations, and beliefs—and energy pirates—the maneuvering and dodging people do to disguise these patterns and beliefs. Recognizing and understanding human energy fields, and how people are sometimes drained by them, is the key to achieving personal and professional fulfillment. Reeder explains how to overcome these personal barriers to heal and create the life of your dreams.

$14.95 • Paper • ISBN 1-58091-048-3

Chakras and Their Archetypes: Uniting Energy Awareness and Spiritual Growth

By Ambika Wauters

Linking classic archetypes to the seven chakras in the human energy system can reveal unconscious ways of behaving. Wauters helps us understand where our energy is blocked, which attitudes or emotional issues are responsible, and how to then transcend our limitations.

$16.95 • Paper • ISBN 0-89594-891-5

Healing Spirits: True Stories from 14 Spiritual Healers

By Judith Joslow-Rodewald and Patricia West-Barker

Photographs by Susan Mills

In an attempt to turn a fantasy into reality, three women, Judith Joslow-Rodewald, Patricia West-Barker, and Susan Mills, traveled across the United States to meet, learn from, and record the stories of practicing healers. These healers' stories and paths are both ordinary and extraordinary, but what they all share is an unshakable belief in the idea that everyone is a potential healer with an innate ability to move toward wholeness.

$20.95 • Paper • ISBN 1-58091-064-5

Inner Radiance, Outer Beauty

By Ambika Wauters

Ambika Wauters encourages women to seek and nurture themselves by dismissing unrealistic images of their bodies. She helps them find their archetype of beauty from within and express their inner awareness by transforming their physical appearance. Includes a 21–day program for regaining health and beauty.

$14.95 • Paper • ISBN 1-58091-080-7

On Women Turning Forty: Coming Into Our Fullness

By Cathleen Rountree

These candid interviews and beautiful photographs will inspire all women who are navigating through the mid-life passage. The updated look of this best-selling classic makes it the perfect companion to the later decades of Rountree's series on women.

$16.00 • Paper • ISBN 0-89594-517-7

Pocket Guide to Hatha Yoga

By Michele Picozzi

Hatha yoga is a holistic form of exercise tailor-made for modern Westerners. This guide offers a roadmap for the beginner and a comprehensive resource for the continuing yoga student.

$6.95 • Paper • ISBN 0-89594-911-3

Pocket Guide to Meditation

By Alan Pritz

This book focuses on meditation as part of spiritual practice, as a universal tool to forge a deeper connection with spirit. In Alan Pritz's words, Meditation simply delivers one of the most purely profound experiences of life, joy.

$6.95 • Paper • ISBN 0-89594-886-9

The Sevenfold Journey: Reclaiming Mind, Body & Spirit Through the Chakras

By Anodea Judith & Selene Vega

Combining yoga, movement, psychotherapy, and ritual, the authors weave ancient and modern wisdom into a powerful tapestry of techniques for facilitating personal growth and healing.

$18.95 • Paper • ISBN 0-89594-574-6

Transforming Body Image: Learning to Love the Body You Have

By Marcia Hutchinson, Ed.D.

Uses step-by-step exercises for self-acceptance to integrate body, mind, and self-image. We recommend every woman read this book.—Ellen Bass and Laura Davis

$14.95 • Paper • ISBN 0-89594-172-4

We are the Angels: Healing Your Past, Present, and Future with the Lords of Karma

By Diane Stein

Stein masterfully presents a detailed understanding of karma and the process of healing karmic patterns. She introduces the Lords of Karma, the supreme karmic record keepers able to grant requests for changed or released karma to those who ask for it.

$16.95 • Paper • ISBN 0-89594-878-8

A Wisewoman's Guide to Spells, Rituals and Goddess Lore

By Elizabeth Brooke

A remarkable compendium of magical lore, psychic skills, and women's mysteries.

$12.95 • Paper • ISBN 0-89594-779-X

Writing from the Heart: Inspiration and Exercises for Women Who Want to Write

By Leslea Newman

There's more to this book than inspiration. For presenting the basics of writing structure and technique, this book has few peers.—Lambda Book Report

$14.95 • Paper • ISBN 0-89594-641-6

Your Body Speaks Your Mind: How Your Thoughts and Emotions Affect Your Health

By Debbie Shapiro

Debbie Shapiro examines the intimate connection between the mind and body revealing insights into how our unresolved thoughts and feelings affect our health and manifest as illness in specific parts of the body.

$14.95 • Paper • ISBN 0-89594-893-1

www.crossingpress.com

BROWSE through the Crossing Press Web site for information on upcoming titles, new releases, and backlist books including brief summaries, excerpts, author information, reviews, and more.

SHOP our store for all of our books and, coming soon, unusual, interesting, and hard-to-find sideline items related to Crossing's best-selling books!

READ informative articles by Crossing Press authors on all of our major topics of interest.

SIGN UP for our e-mail newsletter to receive late-breaking developments and special promotions from The Crossing Press.

WATCH for a new look coming soon to the Crossing Press Web site!